Something On Our Minds

An Anthology to Benefit the Accelerated Cure Project

Volume III

Editors
Laura G. Kolaczkowski
Caroline C. Kyriakou
Sean J. Mahoney
Tracy A. Todd

Something On Our Minds, Vol. III

Printed in the United States

Special Acknowledgements

Many hands and minds worked together on this edition of Something On Our Minds – thanks go out to everyone, but especially the writers who allow us into their view of living with a chronic disease.

The cover art is excerpted from *Brain Fog* by Starr Velez. Starr Velez has lived joyfully with progressive MS. With degrees in psychology Starr is a Life Coach assisting others cope with various diagnoses. She is a veteran, non-profit owner, teacher, established artist, author and global traveler. She lives each moment and finds that nothing is impossible. MS is her blessing and has exposed Starr to opportunities as she continues to consult, teach, volunteer and partake in various sports fulfilling her need for adrenaline and showing that MS or wheelchair does not define her, a smile does.

A special note of thanks to Joker Little, who designed the custom printer's embellishment used in this text. Joker Little is a painter and illustrator from Boston. He helps raise MS awareness with his wife, Caroline Kyriakou, who was diagnosed in 2006.

Table of Contents

A Community of Multiple Sclerosis Organizations i

Introduction to the Accelerated Cure Project iv

Fire Escape 1

After the Seizure, 8/22/13, 1535hrs 3

A Kiss before Falling: The Noir of MS 4

Loss of Independence..8

Senryu Progression 12

Ouroboros 13

A Writer...17

In The Fight Together...18

The MS Walk..19

A Lucky Lady 20

damn legs 26

taking sides...26

A Problem of Faith 27

Borrowed Time 34

Multiple Sclerosis..41

The Broken..42

Invasion 46

Looking Backward....Thinking Forward 47

Interview: Marc Stecker, Wheelchair Kamikaze 52

Footprints and Shadows: The Tao of MS 64

New Beginnings Equal Happier Endings 70

The Dreamer 71

The Survivor's Anthem 72

Solace 73

The Mermaid in the Pool 74

Every Step I Take 79

This Wretched MS and Me 84

I Can Still 85

The Wheelchair Cruise 86

I Went to the Doctor 87

Finding Joy Amongst Pain 90

Rome Wasn't Built In a Day . . .

You Can't Storm the Appian Way 102

Dancing with Multiple Sclerosis 105

Invocation *to Beauty* 116

This Is the Life 118

What Not to Say to Me Now That I Am Crippled 120

Dichotomy of the Tube Slide - A Case Study 122

Decisions, Decisions 136

Portuguese Soup with an MS Twist 141

Cicadas 147

PTSD....................148
Obstacles....................149
If the People Stare, Then the People Stare....................150
Serendipity....................158
Church....................170
Charity Skydive....................173
Interview: Cyndi Zagieboylo....................175
Revelation....................181
Mirror Song....................182
Shy Bear Pass....................183
Nurturing Kids & Fighting Lesions....................185
My Magnificent Spirit....................190
Final Words of Inspiration....................202
Be Part of the Change....................203

From the Editors –

Community of Multiple Sclerosis Organizations

Multiple Sclerosis is a disease of the central nervous system, affecting the brain and spine. It can present in varied ways, but the basic types of MS are Relapsing Remitting (RRMS), Secondary Progressive (SPMS) and Primary Progressive (PPMS). Regardless of the type, people with MS have numerous organizations representing their needs. The Multiple Sclerosis Coalition is comprised of national organizations with a focus on improving the quality of life for people living with MS, as well as researching and finding a cure. Each of these organizations is a trusted and respected resource for the MS community.

The National Multiple Sclerosis Society (NMSS) is an excellent source of information to help understand MS, a chronic and often disabling disease that attacks the central nervous system (brain and spinal cord). Symptoms may be mild, such as numbness in the limbs, or severe, such as paralysis or loss of vision. The progress, severity, and specific symptoms of MS vary among individuals and are unpredictable. NMSS also leads in supporting research for a cure.

Living with MS presents many daily challenges, as noted by the Multiple Sclerosis Foundation (MSF). The quality of a person's life — relationships, education, work, parenting, social activities and more — can be affected by MS. MSF emphasizes that with appropriate symptom management and the ability to adapt, these challenges can be manageable.

That sentiment of empowerment is the centerpiece of another MS leader, Can Do MS. Their philosophy is everything that people who live with this disease and their support partners, is driven by one simple belief: you are more than your MS.

The Multiple Sclerosis Association of America (MSAA) notes that in addition to the treatments that are FDA-approved or in development to limit or slow the MS process, treatments are also being researched for neuroprotection and remyelination, which could potentially return lost function for individuals with MS. The future looks bright as science continues to uncover more vital clues about the immune system and MS. MSAA offers support and services primarily to assist people who might otherwise not have the financial resources.

The International Organization of Multiple Sclerosis Nurses and the Consortium of Multiple Sclerosis Centers offer vital professional development for people in the medical fields for peer mentoring and to stay current on treatment options. These two organizations co-host the largest professional gathering of MS medical specialists in the United States, at their annual convention.

The United Spinal Association (USA) is known for helping paralyzed veterans, but their mission also includes assisting any person with spinal cord injury or damage, including MS, amyotrophic lateral sclerosis and spina bifida. USA leads in the field of advocacy on behalf of the over one million people in the US living with some form of spinal cord disease or injury, as well as the direct one-on-one services they can provide.

The final organization in the MS Coalition is the Accelerated Cure Project (ACP), the recipient of the proceeds from this Anthology. In addition to other research projects, ACP has the support and input from the MS Coalition in the development of a groundbreaking initiative that empowers people with MS to become research partners – iConquerMS™. The leaders of this patient led initiative believe ….

One Person Will Help Conquer MS – YOU!

If you don't already know the Accelerated Cure Project, we are pleased to introduce you to this special non-profit organization.

The Accelerated Cure Project

The Accelerated Cure Project for Multiple Sclerosis (ACP) is honored to receive the proceeds from this volume of *Something on Our Minds.* We work to accelerate the pace of research into the causes, mechanisms and symptoms of MS so that better treatments and lasting cures can be developed and made available.

This anthology was created by many people coming together, contributing their unique talents, ideas and viewpoints to achieve a powerful result. Our work at Accelerated Cure Project follows exactly the same model. We bring together people with MS, doctors and nurses, pioneering scientists, advocacy experts, and many others to accomplish important goals.

MS is a complex disease. Nobody has all of the answers. Only by working together and openly sharing what we have and what we know can we make real progress.

Here are a few examples of how we've harnessed the power of collaboration to accelerate research in MS:

We've brought together people with MS, researchers and clinicians, advocacy groups, and communications and technology experts to create **iConquerMS™**, a network of people with MS contributing data and samples as well as their intelligence and ideas to drive research on topics they care about. Imagine being part of a network where **your** input is valued and **your** ideas about research drive the group's progress. Come and join this network by signing up at iConquerMS.org. Contribute to research on topics that are important to you.

Working with 10 MS clinics, other advocacy organizations, and 3,200 individual participants, we developed the **ACP Repository** to provide much-needed blood samples and data to scientists worldwide. What's so remarkable about freezers full of blood samples and servers filled with data? In the hands of talented researchers, these samples and data have become important breakthroughs in understanding and treating MS. To date the ACP Repository has supported over 90 research studies, exploring topics such as what causes MS and the differences between relapsing and progressive MS. Many of these studies could never have been carried out if not for the repository – but through the power of collaboration, the impossible becomes possible.

In partnership with the MassGeneral Institute for Neurodegenerative Disease, scientific journalists, and researchers worldwide, we provide the **MS Discovery Forum**, an independent, unbiased news and information portal focused on MS research. Just like this anthology, the MS Discovery Forum offers high-quality written material (news stories, features, blogs) to communicate a wide variety of topics to our readers. We also go beyond writing, providing podcast interviews with MS experts and interesting graphic presentations of MS data to enrich the community's understanding of MS. We invite everyone to visit msdiscovery.org to see all that it has to offer.

Accelerated Cure Project applauds all of those who have contributed to "Something on Our Minds," who have shared themselves honestly, openly, caringly to benefit the entire MS community. We strive to do the same: sharing our knowledge and resources honestly, openly, caringly to accelerate research that benefits the entire MS community. We welcome hearing from anyone who would like to get involved in our efforts. Best wishes to all, and thank you for your support.

Hollie Schmidt
Vice President of Scientific Operations
Accelerated Cure Project

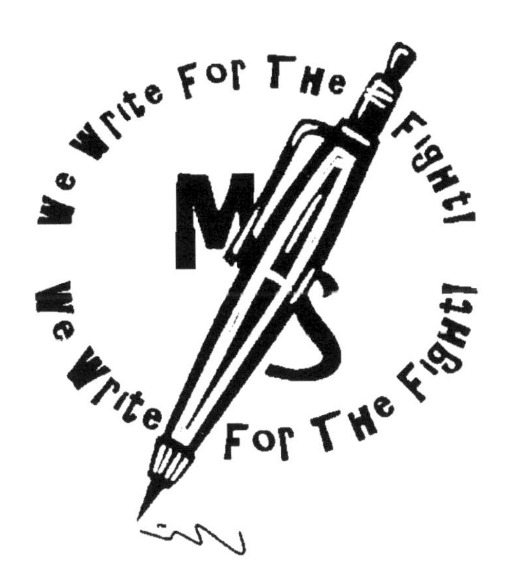

We Write For The Fight™ is an online self-help group founded by Tracy A. Todd. This community welcomes authors and poets with varying degrees of experience and together we share our words to advocate, inform and increase awareness for and about the global MS population.

This dynamic group has published two volumes of "Something On Our Minds" and our journey continues with Volume III ~ An Anthology to Benefit the Accelerated Cure Project.

Contact information: WeWriteForTheFight@gmail.com

Fire Escape

I wish you knew
I was on the pill,
well, many pills
mostly small and white,
here & there an oblong
one, or blue, maybe.

Anyway, I've been
this way since before
I started singing songs.
One day when I was
a kid my legs just
froze and the small
town doctors didn't
know what to do. Of

course my mother prayed—
that might have
been better than the
myelogram or the x-rays
of my head--it was the 70's.
No one could
see into the body

the way they do now.
I've told you of icy dead
fields, where nothing is
greening at all.   Where I go.
Where the hippy kids stretch
on sun-warmed
rocks in February

out in mossy river bottom flow
when the temp climbs
to the 40's in St. Paul,
in a little slip of woods
between the Lutheran
Seminary and the freeway.

I didn't have as much
pain back then. I didn't
know there was a bleak
vaporous space
gathering in my muscles,
my thighs, my abdomen.

Once I was hit
in the head it was over.
I have many words &
memories still flow
like young hot semen.
But the blast of dying
neurotransmitters is controlling
my ropy muscles,
some tendons like glass
or brittle plastic.
Of disorder I can speak
of how the shade becomes
not a reverie but a scene
I can sometimes see
when my sight bends
and my muscles are as granite.
Beyond myself into a world
that exists without me.

–Albino Carrillo

After the Seizure, 8/22/13,1535hrs and Fire Escape are from the book *Uranium Days*, Saudade/Argus House Press, 2015. By permission of author.

After the Seizure, 8/22/13, 1535hrs

No one's here. Only
the cat and the crazy
dogs. Foaming for
attention. For food.
anything wild. And I
am slipping into
the darkness, my
body is glass
my muscles are
like raw wet ropes.
I have not lost
but see only
the darkness in
me gathering
off and on like
violent little thunder
storms. I remain
your friend. But I fear
so much those
episodes of pain
followed by emptiness
eating me alive.

–Albino Carrillo

Albino Carrillo was born in New Mexico. He suffers from Stiff Person Syndrome. He has published two books of poetry, and teaches writing at the University of Dayton.

A Kiss before Falling: The Noir of MS

There is no end to the variety of styles we can use to tell the story of how MS entered our lives. I've always been a fan of noir story-telling, and the darker the better. Most always a thriller, one popular premise is that a stranger comes to town and changes the lives of good and bad folks alike. In noir, the line between them isn't all that clear. The overall tone is fatalistic; everybody is on the same train, nobody can make it jump the tracks and they know it, though most are in denial. They are slaves to their greed or weakness or complacency or fear.

Some noir characters are after something, a thing or an idea, like the Maltese Falcon in *The Maltese Falcon*, or Rosebud in *Citizen Kane*, or diamonds in *The Asphalt Jungle*, or insurance money in *Double Indemnity*. This thing or idea is a plot device that motivates the characters and moves the story forward and is known as a "MacGuffin." The best description of a MacGuffin is uttered by Sam Spade himself in the last line of the *Maltese Falcon*, when Ward Bond asks Humphrey Bogart what the statue is and Bogie responds: "The stuff dreams are made of."

The MacGuffin in our own little noir saga is the cure for Multiple Sclerosis. If you've been paying attention to the buzz in the MS community about the recent influx of new RRMS disease-modifying therapies, you know the volume has gone up considerably on our aggravated grumblings that the research community is knocking out band-aids rather than developing a cure. We are redefining our MacGuffin as being more than a cure, however; it now includes restoration and rejuvenation in the form of nerve damage repair and disability reversal. We are not ashamed to demand more, and why not? It's just the stuff dreams are made of anyway. If we're going to dream, why not dream really, really big?

In Scene One of our little MS noir drama, the stranger that's come to town is Multiple Sclerosis. See how easily some famous crime classics lend themselves to our predicament:

"You were dormant, you were sleeping the big sleep, you were not bothered by things like causing suffering and self-doubt, oil and water were the same as wind and air to you. You just slept the big sleep, not caring about the nastiness of how you would attack or where your victims would fall. Me, I was part of the nastiness now. Far more a part of it than I could have imagined."
— Raymond Chandler from his crime novel *The Big Sleep.*

In the next story, Multiple Sclerosis could be the *femme fatale*:

"He told himself she wasn't really such a bad person, she was just a pest, she was sticky, there was something misplaced in her make-up, something that kept her from fading clear of people when they wanted to be in the clear." — David Goodis, from his novel *Dark Passage.*

And our own story? Let's name this MS noir *A Kiss Before Falling*. The opening scene could go something like this:

That night was like any other that sported a full moon, bright enough to find my way along the narrow unlit side streets of Frisco and dark enough to swathe my face in anonymity, which was an important feature of my nighttime ambling. I was the kind of young thing attracted to shadowy, sad, lonely places and ideas, mostly out of boredom. Nothing much had happened to me. I was too young to be bitter, to have had my heart broken, to have lost everything I owned or lost a loved one to death. I feared loss and at the same time yearned for it. As though that was the only way to build character. To give my life a fresh purpose.

I heard it a split second before feeling it: a crackle, the static electricity kind you hear pulling a comb through your hair on a cold day. It felt like somebody brushed a live wire across my lips just to make me flinch. But I was alone. I flinched all right; my legs crumpled beneath me as though the juice got switched off. My arms hung uselessly at my sides, I couldn't even raise them to protect my face on the way down. I collapsed in a loose heap like a marionette with all the strings cut.

A cloud moved in front of the moon, further darkening the alley where I now lay helpless on the pavement. I thought I'd had a stroke. It wasn't until much later that I learned the name of my stalker: Multiple Sclerosis.

–Kim Dolce

Having taken turns writing for radio and reference books, then cranking out an unbearably serious first novel—Kim Dolce is now exploring the lighter side of life: Coping with MS.

Reprinted with permission. Originally published August 10, 2015 on multiplesclerosis.net.

Loss of Independence

Reading stories about prisoners of war I can imagine that that chapter of their lives must have been a difficult and challenging time.

When I think about a POW in a war I often think about the fact that the person is confined and can't move about like they want to. They are in a strange and unknown place. Often the biggest toll that it takes on the person is the mental one.

I have never been a POW and so I am not writing from firsthand experience. I have read accounts of prisoners of war and I seek to draw parallels between the prisoner of war experience and a person who has MS.

One thing that I learned from the prisoner of war stories, the Diary of Anne Frank, survivors of the Holocaust and stories about slavery is survival and quality of life is about a state of mind. It isn't so much the physical torture or abuse that they endured, but mental torture.

Smart captors know that and they try to get in the prisoner's head. Multiple Sclerosis is much the same way. I often say that unlike a congenital disease where a person is born without sight, hearing or one of the other senses, Multiple Sclerosis robs a person of abilities that they had. The disease inflicts the cruelest kind of torture; loss of independence that the person had before.

My story begins ten years ago when my sons were kids and I would play with them in the backyard. We played football. My sons against dad. I noticed that I couldn't "cut" or change direction quickly when I was running with the football. I went to the doctor and he said, "It's nothing...a lot of people who are in their forties have that problem." I knew that NONE of my friends have that issue. He sent me to a cardiologist. Total waste of money!

I thought that it was vertigo. Meanwhile Multiple Sclerosis was slowly taking my independence. Like a thief in the night, it was quiet and invisible. Unlike a prisoner of war there wasn't any torture. There were questions though. These questions didn't come from a captor. They came from me.

"Why was this happening to me?" The next torture technique occurred while I was walking around the neighborhood with my friend. We usually walked three times a week throughout the neighborhood. We would walk on the sidewalk side by side. I kept veering onto his side one day and he said, "Man, you'd better have that checked out!"

The final torture happened when I went hot-tubbing with a friend of mine one weekend. The heat beat me down and I literally had to be helped out of the hot tub and to the car. I still hadn't been diagnosed so these were unrelated incidents in my mind. I was slowly being robbed... Robbed of my independence. I didn't even realize it at the time.

I went to a different doctor this time. I "fired" the other doctor. The new doctor said he was going to order an MRI. I saw a neurologist at the same clinic and she said that the results of my MRI pointed to several different diseases and the only way they would know for sure is that I have a lumber puncture or spinal tap.

I still hadn't been diagnosed with Multiple Sclerosis, but the thief was in my body! In all of movies that I've seen where they held prisoners of war, the captor would gradually deprive the prisoner of certain things like light, food and clothing.

Multiple Sclerosis is a lot like a captor. It can deprive you of light (optic neuritis), food (loss of appetite) and clothing (heat or cold intolerance).

At the same time that I was having the MRI and the lumbar puncture I was going through another kind of torture. I was going through a divorce. That's another story altogether! I said that I didn't have health insurance when I got the lumbar puncture and the procedure was done gratis by a neurologist in Sugar Land, TX.

I was finally diagnosed April 15, 2010. I began another chapter of my life...

The year that I was diagnosed I call "the year that the wheels came off". I sold my house in Houston and moved back to San Diego, California. Even that process was harrowing! The house was on the market for a while and it finally sold via short sale to a cash buyer. The house was sold and I began to sever all ties with Texas. I quit my job as an adjunct professor at Houston Community College. I farmed out the remaining events that I had on the books to my disc jockey friend in Houston. Life as I knew it was morphing into a shadow of my former life.

One of the things that everyone who has the disease has in common is that we were all very active... uncommonly active.

The loss of independence had begun...

–Marcus I. Brown

Marcus Brown, native San Diegan is a 54-year old father of two sons. Teacher of computer applications. Author. Avid reader. He has come full circle back to his birth place after living in Los Angeles and Houston. Marcus has owned several businesses: professional photographer, mobile disc jockey, etc. Next occupation on his list: successful, published author.

Senryu Progression

Years of MS fears
Why? and What? and How? and When?
And still no answers.

It has been 10 years.
Each day anticipating
Disability.

Why wonder Why? When?
Each day offers a challenge.
Rise up and meet it.

–Carolyn Howard

Carolyn lives in New Hampshire with her husband, 2 beagles and occasionally, some of their 3 grown children and their friends. Diagnosed with RRMS in 2005, she remains fairly active. Over the past few years she, a chemist by training, has chosen to explore more creative areas of her mind.

Ouroboros

The way of multiple sclerosis parallels the stealth of a boa constrictor—muscular, quiet, hidden, coiled around one's brain, opportunistic for the moment it can slide in and swallow your nervous system, part by part, in one long, slow digestive assault.

You try to avoid stress, that favored mantra from the neurologist's office rendered useless in the face of real life, a series of nothing but stressful events, linked by rare pauses in space and time, if one is lucky to enjoy the luxury of remission. MS consumes quality of life, at least, and not quantity, so technically you don't die from it…but that doesn't make it any less sinister.

###

People die, in real life, from all sorts of other unexpected things.

You received the news in a text from your brother just minutes ago. Your mother has died, her brain intact, unlike yours, her body riven by crippling arthritis. Cause of death, respiratory failure, due to pneumonia. Awake, conscious, she succumbed when the morphine exceeded her ability to breathe, and suffocated.

As you surely will do here, in this feed store, despite its high hay lofts and capacity to house a circus.

You tell yourself it is allergies that knot your throat, though you are only sensitive to chemicals and not the floating fibers of straw, the underlying notes of manure. The feed store is a converted barn much larger on the inside than it appears from the road. So much like the lives of the chronically ill.

###

You've come here with her before, to buy cheap pansies and rubberized garden gloves, to pick up your weekly CSA share. The feed store was then, and is still today, a place for breathing, wide open double-high rafters, light shafting through windows open to the sun and bees in reconnaissance, a place bearing the images held close to your mother's from life grown up on a dairy farm.

To think your mother died because she could no longer breathe—despite the longevity of her lung cancer survival at over twenty years—seems improbable. Maybe she, too, carried a secret snake coiled in her chest in hibernation. She had two aunts and two cousins with MS.

Wrapping your brain and heart around this sudden news of her passing renews in you fears both old and recent. It took you years to learn to breathe underwater; only at age forty did you master it without holding your nose. As for the small confinements of your new normal after diagnosis… They never bothered her like they bother you now—the tube of the MRI still requires lorazepam, a washcloth over the eyes, a mother's swaddling of blankets around one's body by the imaging tech, as if to prepare you for your own burial.

You are not sure you will ever get used to any of this.

###

On the bench next to you are packets of bulbs, a mulching fork, a bag of hummingbird nectar you will no longer be able give to her. You hold your breath, hoping the snake doesn't notice. After all, even though you once feared suffocation, your bigger fears, every day, twine around the potential loss of the eyes, the legs, to bladder, and ironically, never the lungs.

It will hit you later, the way your body will absorb this stress, this loss, like poison. The way the boa constrictor waits for the chemical imbalance to unravel nerve fibers, to send inflammation as a flood of tenderizing blood to repair what cannot be fixed.

And behind the rush of this pointless healing: the yawning pink maw of the snake, its only goal to feed on broken places, digesting them whole with potent enzymes in a process stretched over weeks, leaving irreparable the bare spots, the lost functions.

The boa constrictor moves a third of a mile an hour, the same speed in which you process the news now and for months after, grief presenting as the stabbing, vice-like squeeze around the rib cage, called an MS hug, not at all alike the one you wish you could give your mother now.

–Tamara Kaye Sellman

Tamara Sellman is a widely published writer of fiction, nonfiction and poetry, with work nominated for the Pushcart Prize (poetry, fiction) and the John Burroughs Nature Essay Award. She works in sleep technology and education and helps moderate a multiple sclerosis forum. She confirmed her own diagnosis in 2013. www.tamarasellman.com

A Writer

Headache
And fatigue
Attempt to
Prevent me from
Writing these words

I try to make sense
On paper
But the symptoms
Consume me

The pen must
Meet paper

I fight for this

MS will not take this
From me

9 Years and counting
"I have MS
But MS does not have me"

Or does it?

–Caroline Kyriakou

In The Fight Together

When you hear
Someone say
They have MS,

It's an instant
Connection

They understand
The secret struggle

They understand
The invisible disease that
Sneaks up on you

Like a shadow
Always there
But not always seen

And in that instant
You're in the fight together.

–Caroline Kyriakou

The MS Walk

Each step I take
I look around
A sea of orange
Left and right

Friends close
And family closer
They cannot see
The effects each
Step has on me

But they know
I continue on
Step after step

For I
Walk all over MS

–Caroline Kyriakou

Caroline Kyriakou has found a passion for raising awareness for MS since her 2006 diagnosis. She takes pride in participating in Walk MS and was on FOX's Boston morning show in 2010 for World MS Day. Join her Facebook support group: Friends Against the MonSter and follow her at www.facebook.com/CarolineKyriakou.

A Lucky Lady

So I'm sitting on the bench at the playground, watching my youngest son explore in the sand and make a monstrous disaster out of himself, when another mom sits down next to me. This is quite surprising, because she looks well-put-together with her cute little poufy ponytail, adorable pink track suit, and perfectly-applied eyeliner. Her look is completed with a cup of coffee from Starbucks.

Then there's Me: My ponytail is a mass of hyperactive hair, I'm wearing a t-shirt that has at least 4 stains on it, none of which are even the same *color*, my unintentional "raccoon" eyeliner is leftover from yesterday, and I've been in Starbucks a total of 3 times in my life. Generally moms like her look at women like me and figure it's best not to *engage with the animals*, if you get my drift. But there's nobody else around, she's quite pleasant, and I'm game for some conversation.

We chat and share our basic bios, including our professional lives B.K. (Before Kids). I mention I'm not working and I likely won't go back to work again. Wistfully she exclaims, "Oh, you are so ***lucky***!!!" Instantly, my instincts go on the defensive; my insides want to revolt and correct her, to tell her about *my kind* of luck:

I want to tell her that just yesterday, I wrote out another student loan payment check for a bachelor's degree I passionately pursued and completed with honors 15 years ago. It was supposed to be the beginning of my professional development, but instead, it became the last one I'll likely hold. For a person who loves to learn, who valued achieving her independence and relished accomplishment, this is a tough pill to swallow.

I want to tell her that I read voraciously, stay up on politics and study history, and enjoy being a font of useless knowledge, because I've learned that knowing a little something about everything allows me to connect with every individual I meet. I have always loved to exchange ideas, absorb others' life lessons and glean information from intellectuals. But not long ago I'd been "called out" by my sister and best friends for shutting others out of my world; for isolating and becoming reclusive—and they were right. I struggle to track conversations now, and for a lady who never met a stranger, this is a tough pill to swallow.

I want to tell her that not long ago, I had to step back and make a decision about the kind of woman I was going to be, because the one I <u>*intended*</u> to become wasn't going to exist anymore. Cognitively, it simply isn't possible because of the deterioration of my brain and central nervous system; and there were actually tests to prove this wasn't just a paranoid fear—after years of a successful career in pharmaceutical sales, I hadn't even been able to maintain part-time employment at my church and was now on disability. I wasn't a stay-at-home mom because I *wanted* to be, it was because I'd exhausted all options for employment. For a lady who thought the sky was the limit, who prided herself on professionalism and productivity, this is a tough pill to swallow.

I want to tell her that my highest concern is how to raise my 3 sons alone, because my husband of almost 14 years left us last August and our divorce was final a few months ago. Or the unbelievable challenges I faced with obtaining healthcare benefits once he moved out of state; the hours of frustrating phone calls that provided more questions than answers from less-than-helpful government employees. I'm tempted to share the moments each child has collapsed in tears of anguish because of what has happened to our family, when the only comfort I could provide was a mother's love and prayer for their hearts to heal. I could briefly recount the unfair accusations they've hurled at me in their confusion and anger about why their father left, and how it takes all the character I've acquired in my 37 years on earth to answer their questions as honestly as possible while maintaining a position of respect for his role as their dad (regardless of my *personal* feelings). My answer to the standard adult question "What do you do for a living?" is one that makes me speechless now.

Uncomfortable. Grieved. Aimless. For a lady who is starting to pick up the pieces and rebuild her life after assuming it would only be death that parted my college sweetheart from me and our sweet innocent sons, the last two years have been a particularly bitter pill to swallow.

I want to tell her that *luck* has nothing to do with why I'm sitting here next to her on a park bench at 11:00am; that in fact, many people would call me ***un***lucky because of the disease that has threatened my independence and karate-chopped my professional ambitions. It's not easy to depend on someone else for financial security, especially when you're a broad who fully planned to be able to take care of herself from the time she was 15, or feel as though nobody can count on you because you can't remember what you'd promised you'd do anyway.

I *want* to say all those things, except after all these examples of disappointment and life challenges shoot through my brain, they are followed by the faces of the amazing blessings in my life.

Faith, attitude, neighbors, friends, family, and a great sense of humor—all have been essential for me to endure the bitter pill of my losses. Once we've sorted through my sadness and grief together, I can count on God to gently usher me forward to the next groovy assignment He has in mind for me to tackle. And until then, I've been handed the privilege of parenting the 3 most incredibly funny, exhausting, frustrating, brilliantly inspiring boys I've ever met.

So instead, I say, "Yeah... I'm one lucky lady."

–Emily Rhoades

Emily Rhoades is a recovering history nerd, avoidant housecleaner, and eternal optimist. She lives her crazy wonderful life in Peoria, Illinois with her 3 sons, 2 cats, and 1 MS diagnosis. You can follow her blog at lesionedlife.com.

Hunger

I bide my time for hunger.
You too it seems.
While the clatter of cutlery
and chatter of talk
in the kitchen
solicits my attention and grates
against my solitude
like aged dry cheese,
I malinger in my
land of counterpane.
The dinner bell is silent
here and now
while my ears are ringing,
unlike the phone.
Then suddenly the roil of appetite
churns up my belly,
beckons my beggars bowl
to the table
and turns my
aimless quietude to
a cornucopia
of want

–B Milligan

damn legs

your carbonated weakness
fossilized functioning
stone cold indifference

what does it take to
wake you

to take me

–B Milligan

taking sides

here it is
in my littling body
little love
what there is
left
of
right.

–B Milligan

B. Milligan, a Filly of the sixties, a woman of the same years, she had a bittersweet run in the midst of it all. Once married, once divorced, mother of two, lover of the wilds, uncomfortably urban, fixed in time, space and history by circumstance and flesh.

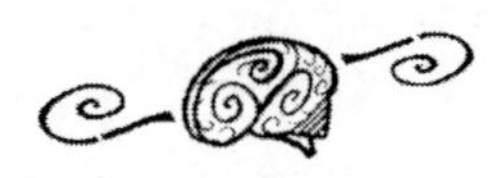

A Problem of Faith

Neurological diseases are a matter of science. They are measurable and they are measured, recipes so nuanced that had they been capable of being reproduced by gifted chefs, it is easy to imagine that Julia Child might have retired much sooner had she bungled early attempts to recreate them at *Le Cordon Bleu.*

Multiple Sclerosis, for example, involves a complex batter of CNS inflammation, brain and spine lesions, axonal degeneration, a certain number of oligoclonal bands, various clinical anomalies, fatigue, phantom pain, optic neuritis. The recipe is not exclusive; other diseases share some of these ingredients. Lyme disease, PML, Transient Ischemic Attacks, Diabetes, bone and blood cancers, atherosclerosis, migraines, Fibromyalgia, thyroid diseases, herpes zoster varicella, Parkinson's. Think of how many recipes use eggs, milk, flour and butter. The light-weight chef might easily set out to make a perfect cheese soufflé and wind up with cheese bread. The dish might look and taste like a soufflé, but only the sophisticated palate of Jacques Pepin could vet this concoction and advise the staff as to whether today's special is *soufflé de fromage* or *pan de fromage*.

The palate of a gifted neurologist can usually vet a cluster of neurological symptoms, evaluate the location and shape of lesions, count the oligoclonal bands in the spinal fluid and compare them to those in the blood serum, review the patient's history of probable flares. The criteria for an MS diagnosis are quantitative as well as qualitative: four o-bands, three lesions, two flares. The degree of disability is measured by numbers on the EDSS, the number of new lesions and their sizes are measured, the number of flares is measured, and the speed of electrical impulses from the eye to the brain is measured. It is science and it is measurable, which suggests that, after a diagnosis is confirmed, it continues to be measurable. And if it is measurable, we assume that the measuring will continue to yield new epiphanies. We assume that these epiphanies will support the narratives we speak to ourselves about how to live.

One narrative is that taking medication will help us live better. The neurologist whose palate identified the sour taste of MS recommends a sweet and protective dressing of disease-modifying therapies. These recipes, too, are science. They are measurable. Their mechanisms have been studied and the dosages have been tested in FDA trials. Interferons, glatiramer acetate, natalizumab, fingolimod. Each has its way of preventing T-cells from damaging myelin. Clinical trials show a 30 percent reduction in relapses compared to placebo. The narrative we tell ourselves is that if we take these drugs then we will have 30 percent fewer relapses. The narrative bespeaks a slowdown in disease progression over our lifetimes. We assume that our improvement will be measurable and that these outcomes will support the narratives we tell each other about how to live well with MS. We do not need to have faith, we have science.

But this is not true.

The more we learn about the therapies, the more gray areas we encounter. Clinical trials, for example, showed a 30 percent reduction in relapses compared to placebo. But this means that the 600 people who took the drug had 30 percent fewer relapses than the control group of 600 people who took a sugar pill. The trial subjects all had a history of at least one flare per year. Their histories of frequent relapses made their outcomes easier to measure.

In real life, we all relapse at various intervals. Our relapse rate on any of the disease-modifying therapies will not reflect that of the trials. If we have a history of relapses that occurred every four or five years, we will have no way of knowing whether the drug is working until many years have passed. We know that relapses follow no particular pattern. The attacks are random. We have no way to measure the number of relapses that might have been had we not taken the therapy. The drug maker asserts no claim that the therapy will actually work at all. If there is a faith narrative within the research community conducting a trial, it is part of the method, the hypothesis that must be tested and then quickly abandoned if the measuring fails to support it.

Science extends no faith narrative to the patient community. Not faith, but rather, hope. We eagerly pick up on the hope narrative. Hope for a cure, new hope for experimental therapy, renewed hope for a cure. We hope that our new therapy will slow the progression and buy us time until there is a cure. HOPE 4 MS is the most common name for MS support groups. Hope can distract us from the breakdown of other narratives. *Taking my medications will make my life better. The more compliant and knowledgeable I become, the better I will be, both physically and emotionally. I'm feeling worse than ever, but I have hope that a better therapy will come along.*

Belief in a higher power offers both hope and faith. Religious narratives are useful and comforting. *If I remain faithful to God, I will be rewarded. I pray to God and he hears me. Doing good will put me in favor with God. I prayed that*

God would restore my vision and after four years of blindness, he blessed me by restoring my eyesight. The most pious among us acknowledge no gray areas. *Your prayers will be answered. If you give yourself to Jesus you will be saved. Tragedies happen for a reason; God wants us to learn something important from them. Evil is always punished; good is always rewarded.*

The positive thinking narrative works similarly. It is the single loudest narrative in American culture. *If I think good thoughts then good things will happen. Stay positive. A happy person is a healthy person. If I believe strongly enough that my cancer will be cured, then it will.* The premise of positive thinking is denial. *I'm going to beat my Stage IV cancer, I don't care what the statistics say. Depression can be avoided if people would just get a positive attitude. I never get sick because I don't believe in disease. It's mind over matter.*

When we speak these narratives to each other and to ourselves, in what, exactly, do we have faith? When our faith breaks down, what is it that makes us fall apart?

The core of our faith is in the belief that our narratives are true. *Ten million people can't be wrong.* We lose our minds when we fear that something we've heard and repeated so many times was only wishful thinking.

The responses to this breakdown are many. Depression, drug and alcohol abuse, suicide. But the majority of us respond with denial. For most of us it is a necessary choice. The devout Christian doesn't abandon her belief in Jesus for very long. Religion is useful and comforting and loopholes abound. *God works in mysterious ways.* Yes, of course, she says to herself, there is so much I don't understand. She begins to feel better, her terror all but forgotten. Many of us can abandon the untrue narrative and embrace a new one, something that might be true. *Copaxone wasn't working after all, I'm going to stop. But Gilenya has a better relapse rate, this might be the one.*

The bravest souls among us are also the boldest. Not only do they abandon the narratives they find false through a crisis, they regularly analyze their narratives and willfully cast out those they feel no longer serve them. They search for no substitutes. They are not unhappy people, only brutally honest. They can live in the moment and say what they observe, knowing that everything could change the moment they finish a sentence. They need no god or hope or platitudes to feel secure. Security itself is a false narrative.

Multiple Sclerosis constantly challenges our life narratives. *Disease happens to other people, not to me. I'm going to be one of that 33 percent of MS patients who will never need a wheelchair. I'm not having a flare, just a bad day. I've had MS for twenty years and never had optic neuritis, so I'll never have optic neuritis. I've taken Avonex for nine years, so this new problem with seizures must have been caused by something else.*

The patient with chronic disease waits for science to catch up with the hope. Whether we embrace, abandon, or modify our narratives is a matter of coping and it is very personal. Our relationship with science is circular; through our life narratives, we maintain our faith that science will triumph, and this brings us hope. Science feeds our hope. The more it advances, the simpler the recipe becomes. *Less is more. This new cancer treatment kills only the abnormal cells.*

The murmur of new MS narratives can already be heard—the rest can be easily imagined. *The MS treatment of the future will be individualized; we'll know the person's bio-markers, her blueprint, if you will, deliver two or three designer molecules to the right spot and presto, she'll run around the block again. It's so simple. Why didn't we see it before?*

–Kim Dolce

Having taken turns writing for radio and reference books, then cranking out an unbearably serious first novel—Kim Dolce is now exploring the lighter side of life: Coping with MS.

Borrowed Time

Like many people with a chronic condition, I will never forget the day a slender, middle-aged physician hovered over me, asking me a series of seemingly useless questions. "Do you do any sort of drugs?" (No). "Have you ever used any type of recreational drugs in your life?" (No). While he was talking, the only thing on my mind was how I needed coffee, and why was this doctor asking me absurd questions at 7:15am? Why was he even in the hospital at 7:15am? I tried to glance up towards him and at least pretend like I was listening, but instead I was nearly blinded by the fluorescent hospital lighting. It's early! Why do they have to keep the lights so bright in here?

Then he said something that I heard loud and clear: "You have Multiple Sclerosis. There is no cure, but there are several treatment options available to prevent the progression of the disease. Due to the depth and frequency of your lesions, I suspect you've had this for a long time, and at this rate, you will need a cane by 28, and a wheelchair by 30."

To avoid looking at him, I glanced down, only to notice I was wearing an MS Walk t-shirt; it's one of my favorite shirts, and I wear it often to bed. I had participated in the MS Walk numerous times in the past, and wearing the shirt was just a sick irony in this scenario. I was only 23 years old, and about to begin my journey of medical school applications. How could I ever become a doctor when I may need a cane during morning rounds? The only person who can pull that off is Dr. House; the real world isn't quite as kind.

"I know you're contemplating medical school, but please don't forget, you can file for social security disability, as you might struggle to find employment."

Those words echoed in my head literally for years. My initial thoughts were much more graphic in nature, and my first thought was to say, "Who do you think you are automatically saying I won't ever become a doctor, or I won't be employable in any type of career? I don't take rejection very well, and I'm certainly not going to be demoralized by some skinny doctor who probably has no friends."

After he left my room, I picked up the phone and called my parents. Growing up with a mother as a physician and a father as a graduate school professor, not obtaining a higher education was never an option. When I received my college diploma, I was elated because I had graduated with a double major, in two very different disciplines, and was pleased with my achievement. As a graduation present, my mother handed me an expensive piece of jewelry and simply said, "You'd better have a career plan that includes professional school because a bachelor degree will not be the end."

How on earth was I going to explain that I had MS, and that, according to my doctor, professional school or any sort of respectable career may never happen? My father received his doctorate in social work, so I already knew he would have no knowledge of what multiple sclerosis is, or how it's contracted. How on earth was I going to explain this to him?

My father arrived at the hospital within a half hour, holding a bouquet of my favorite flowers. Despite his anxiety, he tried to assure me that everything would be okay, and we'd do everything humanly possible to beat this. He requested to see the doctor, who quickly came back to answer any questions my father may have. I had the pleasure of hearing the diagnosis again, discussion of social security benefits, and of course, and the bleak prognosis. Shortly thereafter, my father and I left the hospital. We walked to the car slowly, and didn't say more than one word the entire car ride home.

My mother was waiting when we got home. She couldn't look at me, or say anything either. It was almost as though both my parents weren't particularly concerned about the immediate effects, but rather, what this all meant for my future. Over time, I learned that my future was more about perceptions from others instead of my future with regards to this disease.

I spent the next year of my life undergoing numerous hospital visits for second, third, fourth, and even fifth opinions, IV steroids, and a frequent customer card at Friendly's since ice cream was the only thing that didn't taste awful. Every morning, I would wake up, and gently set my feet on the floor to see if I could stand up properly. This was followed by a self-vision assessment: Could I see? Was everything blurry? Once those two were completed, I would try to find the lowest frequency I was able to hear. I would play the radio at the lowest volume simply to see if I could hear it. It was almost as though I was testing myself; daring myself to prove that I could beat MS.

As the years progressed, I struggled with two spinal taps, a job in retail, and community service. I volunteered at a local emergency room, and realized that my passion for healthcare was stronger than ever. It brought me an indescribable happiness to watch patients come in with an ailment and walk out with some sort of solution, even if it wasn't the best answer. I found myself wondering if these people were also thinking like I was? We are all just borrowing time because the end is inevitable. As my desire to pursue my career became more apparent, I began to wonder if I was on borrowed time, did I really want to spend that brief time with my head in textbooks that weighed more than a small child?

After more considerations, I realized that I did want to pursue my career in medicine because it was the only thing that genuinely interested me, and provided me with a profound sense of contentment. I began my applications, and was accepted to a medical school, even though my resume had been somewhat vacant for a few years.

My first day, I met people who would eventually be my colleagues. I realized immediately these people were not there to be friendly, or even be empathetic, as we were all shooting for the same thing: a career as a doctor. I kept my diagnosis as private as possible. However, given the small nature of the school, and my monthly absences when I was getting my infusion therapy, malicious rumors began. "OMG! Did you hear? She has some sort of disease that requires her to leave class for a day EVERY MONTH! She's never going to make it through med school, I mean you can't even skip a beat in this career." Or, "What is this girl thinking? I heard she has multiple sclerosis! She won't be able to walk, and we all know she has a tremor, I mean, have you seen her in the anatomy lab? It's clear surgery is out."

I heard these things and did my best to not let them affect me. Like anything else, they would sting, but I was blessed when I actually told the Dean of my school about my situation. He stopped everything he was doing, looked me straight in the eye and said, "I know a lot of people are going to give you a hard time, but don't you dare give up. You have a lot of potential, and I know you can do this. I believe in you." Upon hearing that much needed encouragement, and having a proverbial Hallmark moment, I made it through Basic Science (the classroom part of medical school) without failing any classes, or missing any infusions. Without hearing those words from someone whom I respected dearly, I would have never been able to get as far as I have. Fortunately, I'm now blessed to be able to call him my professor, my mentor, and my friend.

So where does all this leave me? I'm still borrowing time because my thirtieth birthday was a long time ago, and I do not have a cane or a wheelchair. The training wheels have been officially removed, and I am actively studying for the first part of the licensing exam. It's hard. Very hard. But do I think I'm unable to finish what I started? Absolutely not. Apart from studying, what else do I do with my limited time? I keep track of all my medications, and if there are any new treatments available. I had some unfortunate luck with the oral medicines, and had to switch to a chemotherapeutic agent, and digesting that emotionally has certainly been difficult, but I'm well aware that it needs to be done. I'm not too fond of the insane fatigue that occurs immediately after the infusion, but fortunately, it wears off rather quickly. Daily, I remind myself that my career decision was my choice, and that I am on borrowed time. I should be elated to have the opportunity to do something I love, and also because, thus far, my initial prognosis hasn't come true. I am still walking without a cane, and at 31 years old, I do not see a wheelchair in my immediate future.

In essence, the purpose of my writing this article is to remind every person out there with Multiple Sclerosis, or any other limiting disease, that these conditions are nothing more than limitations, but are not climactic. With hard work and dedication anything can be accomplished. If someone tells you otherwise then they have no business being in your life. We all know that life is short; why not spend it doing what you love, and with people you love? All of us need to remember that one day, someone will find a cure for this insidious disease, and until then, we need to hang on. Keeping in mind that as of right now, we are all on borrowed time, we need to be optimistic that someone (far more intelligent than me) will find a cure. Hope sustains life. We've all had hope during this borrowed time, so what is the harm in hoping for bigger and brighter things?

–Nidhi Suri

Nidhi Suri is 31 years old. Medical student. Global denizen. Apart from spending her time studying, she enjoys reading, spending time with family & friends, traveling, shopping, and volunteering.

Multiple Sclerosis

My life has changed dramatically.
Unfamiliar sensations invade my body.
Little by little I lose control of what I was, but
To give in to this disease is not an option.
Independence is what I treasure; even as it is
Pulled away from me with each new relapse.
Legs, which were once strong, are now
Erratic in function and form.

Symptoms may change my lifestyle but not my
Courage to stand my ground and fight this battle.
Lightning bolt jabs, fatigue and muscle cramps are part of my
Ever changing body.
Regrets for what is lost, are not an option
Only a sense of choosing a middle ground to
Stand and fight this disease that
Invades my body and mind,
Surrender will never happen as I have MS but MS does NOT have me.

–Brenda Tierman

Past endeavors include Nurse Paralegal, Co-Leader on MedHelp.org MS Community and private contractor for a pharmaceutical company. Brenda Tierman is a Lead Patient Advisor on an MS research project and involved in MS and disability advocacy. She advises on the MedHelp.org forum as time allows.

The Broken

He floats in the rafters at Wal-Mart near clusters of lost Get Well balloons, looking down on the swastika shape of himself in one of the wide aisles arranged for the selling of random crap. How he ended up in Wal-Mart—out of body—is anybody's guess. His last wisp of memory places him behind the wheel of his truck driving through a fog. His fog.

The fog's not here now, above or below.

The rafters are bright industrial ice caves washed in droning artificial light. Fourth of July sparklers crackle across the expanse of his scalp, popping and snapping like the crush of cellophane.

Fucking fluorescent tubes…but this is Wal-Mart. No cure for it.

He simultaneously feels the cold floor pressed against the cheek of his earthbound twin. The unswept lint of the floor feels like pea gravel embedded into his skin. He feels grounded, and not.

# # #

From this lookout, he surveys the grid of the store: gray tiled roads trafficked by the Broken. The obvious ones gain ground on tennis-balled walkers. Others rub their eyes as if blindness can silence the owl wings batting against the decayed walls of their minds. Someone sneezes a comet of green into a bin of cheap yarn.

And he can smell the odor of another's failed bone marrow even from here.

He knows about broken. Multiple sclerosis. No cure for it, either.

People collect about his body like moss, and just as inactive. He feels his blood, even from above, ooze like lava through his body, pulsate and orange, yet cooling to silver at an alarming rate.

Call her! He watches his own eyes blink. *Now!* He watches the hand nearest his jacket pocket slowly withdraw the phone.

He blanks. How to unlock it?

A sparkler burns across the back of his skull in a straight path that terminates at the center his forehead: memory retrieved.

# # #

I'm at Wal-Mart. I've had a fall.

Her voice asks questions he has little fuel left to process.

I'm in the aisle where they sell the random crap.

Dial tone.

A middle-aged slob in a rockabilly haircut and blue apron asks nobody in particular what happened.

I saw him standing there and then his knees just buckled—

—and then, by some miracle of compressed time, she appears, still wearing her sunglasses. It is never foggy for her.

# # #

Did nobody call 9-1-1?

The people around her are lucky they cannot see the death rays in her eyes, he thinks.

She bends down, says his name, the sound of her voice a silver guitar string reuniting twins, rafter and tile.

Sparklers fizzle. He falls back into himself, adrenaline thinning venous sludge, his heart asserting its rhythm. His bones scream from deep inside their wells. He tethers to his reflection in her lenses, grateful.

She has been, will always be, his road crew—filler of potholes when the pavement fails him.

He hears spoken words behind them but he can't process their meaning, though she is quick to interpret. *He's sick, you stupid fuck!* Before the useless and inanimate crowd, she spatulas him off the floor.

He leans into the dam-like strength of her shoulder, shuts his eyes against vertigo, and finds himself privately screening the last film in his memory: he'd walked these aisles banked in fog, wondering numbly how he'd gotten there, and then tripped on some crack in the tile. It may as well have been the Grand Canyon. Man down.

He's too young to be sick, crows an old woman in a velour track suit.

It is easier to not reply. There are no longer sparklers, but lightning bolts that zap his chest, his knee, his cheek. Strange tangible relief. A headache swells into place, the last threads of his cognitive fog floating to the rafters, flocking the countless ghosts of the Get Well party.

The rockabilly clerk snickers. *He's not sick, he's drunk.* Dismissive laughter as the crowd dispels.

He shakes his head *No* when she tenses to strike back. What is the use? No cure for that, either.

–Tamara Kaye Sellman

Tamara Sellman is a widely published writer of fiction, nonfiction and poetry, with work nominated for the Pushcart Prize (poetry, fiction) and the John Burroughs Nature Essay Award. She works in sleep technology and education and helps moderate a multiple sclerosis forum. She confirmed her own diagnosis in 2013. www.tamarasellman.com

Invasion

I had a very bizarre dream before waking this morning and could not make rhyme nor reason of it until I had a chance to mull it over a bit:

I was standing in the yard by the back steps when I noticed a swarm of wasps crawling all over the house where the shingles met the foundation. There must've been an area a foot high by 6-8" wide that was solid with wasps and an additional area surrounding that spot where the wasps were thinning but still very active. Then a large mouse began to crawl up the side of the house and the wasps started attacking it, stinging it thousands of times while it clung to the side of the house for dear life. Suddenly it was raining and the wasp attack was so vicious that it had penetrated the electrical wire going up the side of the house causing it to short out in the rain and now in addition to being stung mercilessly, the mouse was also being electrocuted. Then... the mouse was lying charred and dead in a puddle of water. The wasps seemed to have gone but the side of the house was charred and the shingles blackened and unrecognizable.

My MS has been making itself known for the week in a more consistent and tangible way than ever before. Even with medication, I am so exhausted by midday that I can hardly function. My left leg has felt like it was asleep from 10 or 11 o'clock on, I am starting to trip over my foot, my vision is going and my bladder is not working right. I am the corner of the house (or maybe I'm the mouse... or both) and I have tickling wasps walking all over me and sometimes stinging and incapacitating me so much that the electrical circuitry is damaged. My body is being invaded by unwelcome pests.

–Cherie Binns

From October 1995

Looking Backward....Thinking Forward

Today is a day of change, of epiphany, of growth, of release, of surrender. For weeks now, I've been doing as told in the healing regimen and have been letting the message of **dis**-ability and future decline play with my psyche. I do not, in my very core of being, believe that the therapy course that I have been following since January 25th (75 days) is right for ME or working on my behalf! The job now is to decide whether it's the devices and how they are used that are wrong or whether it is my understanding of the routine, self-image or less than complete mental surrender that is where the problem lies.

I went for my massage this morning and told John some of my struggle and I and targeted areas that needed physical work. Almost as soon as the massage got underway, I began to pray…

Lord, show me your way. Make known to me the path you have for me to travel. Teach me what I need to know to move forward.

I saw a huge vista before me from a great height. It was immediately clear that it was the path of my journey starting in a low fertile land near the shore. The road was initially (and for some distance) straight and free of visible obstacles. But there were dips in the road as I traveled and the pavement was not always smooth. Then the road veered sharply to the right as it approached a steep rock face over which poured a waterfall forming a surging river at the base of the rock. The water was so big and forceful that there was no safe opportunity to cross for a very great distance so the road detoured for many, many miles and over a great deal of time before continuing in yet another direction and up a rocky incline. Vegetation thinned.

The terrain appeared harsh and unforgiving, but from my vantage point much higher, I could tell that the distance had been covered and I had left that rough place behind as well. I was so far beyond it I could not see the path that had brought me to this height. **<u>But</u>** I could see that the path I was traveling did not appear to lead me back to the place I'd begun this journey.

And here, I thought I was rehabbing to return to pre-injury baseline. It must be true that we can't go back!

As I surveyed this "journey vista", it dawned on me that this was not a trip I'd have willingly chosen but was one that, amazingly, I'd been pretty successful on to this point having climbed over great obstacles and expended enormous amounts of energy to be looking back on all of this. (Here it must be noted that my "vision" only extended in the direction from which I had come and I did not see where I have yet to travel… nor did I attempt to.)

As the end of the time on the massage table approached, my thoughts turned to the qualities within that had allowed me to travel this distance:

- Inner drive
- A sense of direction
- Fortitude
- Conviction
- Discipline
- Obedience
- Honesty (I don't cut corners in the therapy plan)
- Desire

- Persistence
- Patience

Then…a new idea emerged in the prayer path that had paralleled the body work. *"Lord, I know if you touched my foot, it would be healed. I do have faith. I believe. I bow to your will for me knowing you want only the best for one you love so deeply."*

Rather than finishing the massage with Reike to my face or neck as is his routine, John sat and took my left foot gently and firmly between his hands and I KNEW Jesus was honoring my request.

I shared all of this with John as we were making up the massage bed for the next client. He chuckled, shook his head, and I think both of us choked up a bit.

"When I started your massage, I asked God not only to show me how to best minister to the needs of your body, but to speak to your spirit about the need to affirm your gifts and strengths. I asked Him to show you how far you'd come, the obstacles you'd overcome without giving in to defeat, and to focus on your strengths for the journey still ahead." Regarding the Reike on the foot…

"I just had a **very clear** directive to do Reike on your foot…something I've never done and would not normally do."

I have been touched by God today and healing has moved to a different level.

–Cherie Binns

(from April 10, 2006)

Cherie Binns, RN BS MSCN, was diagnosed with MS in 1994, after 20 years of episodic symptoms. She became a registered nurse in the 1970's and earned her MS Clinical Nurse certification in 2003. Her writing reflects her experiences with MS and its treatment.

Interview: Marc Stecker, aka Wheelchair Kamikazee

SOOM reached out to blogger Marc Stecker, aka The Wheelchair Kamikaze, and asked a few questions about his blog and specifically the "Footprints and Shadows: The Tao of MS" piece from October 2009 as it seemed to beckon SOOM.

WK: I'm kind of glad you chose the "Footprints and Shadows" essay. It's long been one of my favorites, and I've had long time blog readers tell me that it's a "go to" essay for them to read when they start feeling lost. I've often reread it myself during turbulent times. Funny, reading things that you wrote years ago, they sometimes seem to have been written by some other person…

SOOM: You wrote then that "my efforts to battle the illness are best born from tranquility and quiet determination, and not from the turmoil of desperation." So I am curious if you still approach MS in this way or if time and increased disability has weakened your resolve.

WK: Great question. I definitely continue in my attempts to take a focused and controlled approach to battling my disease, but as the disabilities mount and the complexities and questions surrounding my illness multiply it becomes harder and harder to not simply grab desperately at any strands of hope that present themselves. However, I long ago learned that one should never let hope eclipse reason, and that goes for all of life, not just battling disease or other hardships. Hope is a vital element propelling forward every human endeavor, but in the face of the fear and horror that the prospect of "dark of the end of the MS tunnel" can bring, I think it's vitally important to try not to let oneself flounder and succumb to the irrational. I suppose at times a shotgun approach to trying to fight the disease may in fact prove effective, but I tend to think that it's the sniper who more often hits his bull's-eye, especially if the target is stealthy and difficult to identify. I think the key is "selective aggression", a concept I came to fully appreciate at the poker table…

SOOM: Interesting you use the battle motif. I wrote an essay recently and mused about aggression and MS. I tried applying a gender to the beast but concluded that it too easily fit both the male archetype of warrior (usurper/barbarian) and female archetype of femme fatale (mystery/indifferent). Either way it is in this thing to win at all costs.

WK: Yes, the disease is a formidable adversary. All forms of MS can be hellacious, but the progressive forms of MS, which continue to defy almost all attempts at treatment, are especially daunting. I don't mean to minimize the struggles of the folks with RRMS, who have to deal with the constant uncertainties that go hand-in-hand with having a relapsing remitting disease, but I can only speak of what I know. Having now dealt with the constant grinding progression of progressive MS for 12 years, it's hard not to see this as a battle of attrition. Despite having lived through it, it seems almost unfathomable to me that 12 1/2 years ago I was relatively symptom-free, though I'd had an inkling something was wrong for quite a few years leading up to the "day of the limp", when my disease decided to make itself clearly evident. Suddenly, the line between healthy and sick had been crossed, and things would never again be the same. Still, even then, I had no idea the physical toll the illness would exact. The psychological impact of watching oneself disappear by inches can't be overstated, and the tools and perspective provided by Eastern philosophy, which I talk about in "The Tao of MS", have proven vital in navigating the emotional minefield that accompanies the physical fight.

SOOM: I realize that this is sort of a generic question but do you think that living in NYC – loudest of the loud, more bombast for your buck – has brought a greater clarity to the teachings of Zen Buddhism and Taoism?

WK: Funny enough, although I spent my childhood and teenage years in NYC, and then my college days and first years of my young adulthood in Boston, it was while I was living in Florida that I turned to Eastern philosophies. Through a strange set of circumstances, when I was about 26 years old I found myself an accidental resident of South Florida, a place I never much liked and definitely never intended to live. At that point in my life I was "at ends", as they say, and didn't have much choice in the matter. I was a stranger in a strange land in that place, even though I somehow managed to stay there for a decade. I never fully integrated into the S. Florida way of life, and soon enough found myself living an existence for which I was by temperament ill-suited. The inner turmoil that this disconnect between who I was at my core, and where and how I was living is what ultimately sent me looking for some kind of psychological and philosophical grounding. And though I began reading and studying Eastern philosophy at that time, it wasn't until MS struck (after I had moved back to NYC) that I was able to fully incorporate many of the tenets of the teachings into my daily existence. More out of survival instinct than anything else, really. The shock of having to face down a chronic progressive illness made real some of the abstractions of Eastern thought, and they became my life raft…

SOOM: Example?

WK: Well, the Eastern philosophies all emphasize that there is no such thing as an inherently "good" or "bad" occurrence, it is through our thoughts and perceptions that we experience moments as such. And since with practice we can control our thoughts and emotions, we can shape our own realities. Not that you can turn something like MS into a "good" thing, but in reality it's just a thing in a life made up of a series of things, each of which we assign meaning through the filter of our thought processes. At the heart of Buddhist thought is the notion that all life is suffering, suffering brought on by our attachments to desire, and the things we desire, be they people, physical objects or psychological abstractions. By letting go of those attachments we can reduce our suffering. MS has forced me to relinquish attachments to many things, both physical and psychological. I used to love driving little sports cars, now I don't think I could even get into one. I avidly collected antique wristwatches, and now I couldn't wind one or strap one to my wrist without great difficulty. I chased a version of success that I never fully embraced, wandering further and further from the path I once thought I would follow. Eastern thought stresses the folly of vanity, and it's awfully hard to be vain when one half of your body is withered and useless, and your backside is stuck in a wheelchair. In many ways MS has forced me to live an ascetic life, shedding the trappings of "success" along the way, much as Siddhartha renounced the material wealth and privilege of his royal upbringing. Not that I mean to compare myself to the Buddha, the only thing we might have in common is a big round belly — mine courtesy of years spent sitting in a wheelchair - and perhaps a shared sense of the absurdity of it all…

SOOM: Well we should all aspire to the belly anyway. So this will be pure conjecture but how do you think the Taoist Masters would react (or not react) to stem cell therapy(s)?

WK: I'm sure the Taoist Masters would jump at the chance to partake of a truly effective stem cell therapy, but wouldn't force the issue or allow themselves to succumb to the siren song of some of the less than honest folks hawking miracle treatments to the desperate. The words "stem cells" have become almost magical in their power, but the reality is that, at least in terms of treating MS, the science of stem cells is in its very early infancy. That said, there are some forms of stem cell therapy that are more mature, such as HSCT for RRMS, which certainly warrant serious consideration. Though the Taoist stress "action through inaction", they also stress the importance of clarity of thought and not letting emotion cloud decision-making. Quieting the mind to allow oneself to hear the whispers of the universe is vital, just as it's vital for MS patients to try to cut through the clamor surrounding stem cells and recognize what is real and what is hype, and to then act accordingly.

SOOM: One of the things I've enjoyed most about your blog, Marc, is the intra-connectedness of the entries; it's as if you have opened all of the doors and windows and portals in this 350-room mega-mansion that happens to also be your head. There is an overwhelmingly strong conversational sense to your style. I've never felt uneasy regardless of how deeply scientific or personal the subject matter. It seems like I am in one of the outtakes from My Dinner with Andre you know? Is that deliberate?

WK: Well, I think much of the conversational nature of the blog is due to the fact that because of my disabilities I use voice recognition software to dictate my posts, so, in fact, they really are the result of a very one-sided conversation. I started the blog with very little understanding of what a blog even was. Wheelchair Kamikaze originally was intended to be a place simply to park my photos and videos someplace on the Internet where friends and family could easily access them. As the emphasis shifted to writing, though, I decided that there was no point to putting on pretenses, and I've always been someone who wears his heart on his sleeve anyway. Of course, we are all multifaceted personalities who show different sides of ourselves to different people under different circumstances, so the Wheelchair Kamikaze me is certainly not the whole picture, but I do try to cut through all the bullshit and get to the heart of the matter, whether I'm talking about medical research or more personal subjects. There's something cathartic about bearing the soul, and while we all have our secrets, I suppose the blog does serve as a confessional of sorts. But, believe me, if folks could see me sitting around in my shorts watching deliciously bad 50 or 60-year-old movies I'm sure it would add some depth to their perception of the real me…

SOOM: Are you talking boxers or Bermudas? Movies like Thunder Road?

WK: Ha, most often would be boxers, and I'm talking about lots of old Godzilla movies and the "B" movies of the 30s, 40s, and 50s. Which, in my opinion, are actually much better than a lot of the "A" movies of today… You watch old films and realize that at one point not all that long ago the major studios actually put out movies for adults. Our entire society has been dumbed down to the point where comic books are now the inspiration for our most popular films. The decline of civilizations… Even Godzilla, the original, had some very serious undertones. Not that I'm against a little escapism every once in a while, but it seems that escapism has become the name of the game…

SOOM: I'm curious if, at times, this "baring the soul" seems like a type of performance art? An all too vivid version of life imitating art imitating art imitating hot dogs imitating light and dark...

WK: Like I said, even at my most open, I'm only baring parts of myself, as much of me remains a mystery to me. Is it even possible for a person to truly bare their soul? I think we are always discovering new and unexplored parts of our souls, and writing the blog has helped me shine a light on some of the harder to reach nooks and crannies of my own. Some of the things lurking in those nooks and crannies have been priceless, like rediscovering relics of my childhood personality left untouched by the warping influences of adulthood, but others are definitely better left undisturbed. As far as art imitating life for life imitating art, who the hell knows? Eggplant armpit fried eggs vexing genuflecting marsupials, you know what I mean?

SOOM: Um…yes…yes of course I know about fried marsupials vexing eggplants. Doesn't everyone? If not then everyone should get the red vinyl edition with 3D-glasses. What is the voice recognition software you use and is it available cross-platform?

WK: I use Dragon NaturallySpeaking, by a company called Nuance. I'm on Windows, but the software is available cross-platform. I think the Apple version of the software is called Dragon Dictate, if I'm not mistaken. I'd highly recommend it to anybody experiencing trouble typing, and that goes for people with MS or not. I wish I'd discovered the software in my healthy days. I always hated typing and it's a blast watching your words just appear on the screen as you say them…

SOOM: Can we talk for second about the Garbage Lady photograph on the WK site. There are a lot of great shots there but this one in particular strikes me as very emblematic of the MS struggle: the questions, the unknown, the crap, the reluctance, and perhaps even resignation. Can you talk about the when and where of the picture?

WK: That shot was taken in one of the large, public outside areas at Lincoln Center. I've always been fascinated with people and can people watch for endless hours, though these days I often find myself battling a terrible envy for all of those whose bodies haven't failed them, and who simply don't realize how lucky they are. But there I go, flying off on a tangent. I'm not really sure what the "Garbage Lady" was exactly doing, and since it was shot on the fly during the day I took dozens of photos, I didn't realize quite what I had captured until I came home and started looking through that day's haul. Was the lady hiding from somebody, looking for something, or did I simply capture an awkward moment that had no context whatsoever? I hadn't really thought of the photo as being emblematic of MS, but rather as an example of the fact that people can find themselves in the strangest of situations due only to the vicissitudes of the moment. I'm sure that woman would be mortified to know that she was captured for posterity in that particular pose, however fleeting it was. Who knows, 15 seconds later she may have looked positively elegant, but in that instant she nicely sums up the absurdity of life, and life with MS is, among many things, absolutely absurd.

SOOM: The tangents are, in many instances, part of the charm of The Wheelchair Kamikaze. Just my opinion of course. Maybe the Garbage Lady would take umbrage but unless she comes forward to make her case...

WK: I'd say without hesitation that the tangents are the most interesting things in life. What's that old cliché: life is what happens while you're making plans? As for The Garbage Lady, I'd hope that the thing she would take most umbrage to is the fact that we've now labeled her "The Garbage Lady". Not a flattering moniker…

SOOM: Definitely not…her people will contact you when the time comes. Maybe emblematic is too strong. I was struck the first time I saw her by how summary the composition of the photo was: how did I get here and what the hell am I doing here and who else is watching me here now...right now? MS just chaperoned me to that precise sliver of time.

WK: Yeah, that shot is just a frozen moment, just like any other photograph. I suppose that's the appeal of Street photography, capturing momentary realities in a sliver of light and dark. The iconic photographs manage to capture more than that, though, somehow presenting universal truth to the viewer in the form of a soulful glance or agonized moment, fleeting in reality but stamped with a permanence by the photographer. I once read an essay written by a woman who was shocked to see her own crying visage in a magazine, snapped by a photographer who somehow caught her in a distraught public moment following some upsetting episode in her life. She felt violated, but having expressed her emotions in a public place there was nothing she could do to protect her privacy. And in the end the incident she was so upset over was but a passing chapter in her life. As Kipling once wrote 'Triumph and Disaster are both imposters'.

Many members of supposedly primitive tribes forbid having their pictures taken, fearing that capturing their image also captures a part of their soul. I think they may be right, but that's the point, isn't it?

SOOM: Vulture culture. Anyway - let's throw some humor into the final mix. Here is a joke that my nephew came up with when he was 5-ish (he's 8 now): "Why was the poor boy sad?

Because he didn't have any strawberries." And I will follow that with two Knock-knock jokes that have no origin story I am aware of...in fact I think Knock-knock jokes are really eternal beings literally captured and confined within corniness. So if...Knock-knock. Who's there? Amos. Amos who? A mosquito....then...Knock-knock. Who's there? Anna. Anna who? Another mosquito. Do you have any jokes?

WK: Why did the monkey fall out of the tree? Because it was dead… What's the weather report for Mexico City? Chili today, hot tamale…

SOOM: Cool! Thank you Marc. Truly appreciate you making the time for us.

SOOM Interview was conducted by Sean Mahoney

Footprints and Shadows: The Tao of MS

Getting MS was never on anybody's agenda. None of us ever planned on getting sick, and the shock of the diagnosis is an uppercut to the jaw, a stunning blow that knocks some patients off balance forever.

During the never-ending process of learning how to spiritually and psychologically deal with my progressing disability I've found great solace in the Eastern philosophies of Zen Buddhism and Taoism. These philosophies emphasize that we each create our own reality through our perceptions and emotional responses to all that happens around and to us. Since our emotions are born of us, and not we of them (as popular culture would have us believe), we have the power to create our own happiness despite whatever circumstances life throws at us, by exercising control over those emotions. Nothing that happens to us is inherently "good" or "bad", it is our perceptions and reactions to the goings-on of existence that define them as such.

This is not an easy concept to grasp, let alone put into practice, especially when you find yourself experiencing "creeping paralysis" (an actual early medical term for Multiple Sclerosis), but the only way to avoid utter despondency and hopelessness in the face of such a predicament is to mindfully and willfully refuse to define whatever obstacles life challenges you with as miserable. Happiness is a conscious choice that must come from within, and those who rely on outside sources as their fount of happiness are doomed to a life of perpetual discontent.

In fact, we live in a society that has evolved to deliberately breed dissatisfaction. Discontent fuels our economy; we're constantly bombarded by messages telling us that our problems can be solved through consumerism, that they stem from the fact that our teeth aren't white enough, our possessions – no matter how plentiful – are somehow lacking, and that popularity and sex appeal can only be attained by drinking the right beer or using the latest breakthrough in armpit deodorants. The true meaning of success is a BMW, sexual fulfillment awaits those who don the right pair of Levi's, and self-worth can be found in a really cool pair of Nikes. Happiness is equated with physical beauty, and the modern mythology of movies and television indoctrinates us with the belief that others can "complete" us and bring fulfillment that in reality can only come from within. This search for identity in romantic attachment has led to a divorce rate of over 50%, and instead of bringing everlasting happiness breeds a perpetual state of dissatisfaction we often feel for both our mates and ourselves.

It's incredibly easy to be seduced by these messages when you're healthy and striving to attain some preordained definition of success, even if you consider yourself enlightened and aware of the efforts being made to seduce you. Before I was forced to the sidelines by MS I made my money by playing a part in manufacturing these illusions, and still I was susceptible to them.

Once chronic illness hits, though, it's as if a veil of delusion is ripped away, and blindness abruptly gives way to vision. Suddenly, the absurdities of these notions of consumerist contentment come into crystal view. My physical condition won't allow me to drive a BMW, or any automobile, for that matter (and I was a guy who loved driving, zoom, zoom), fumbling with the button-down fly of the hippest pair of ridiculously expensive jeans would soon find me peeing in my pants, and unless those Nikes can somehow make my legs work again, they just aren't gonna do me any good. Still, such messages are beguiling, siren songs that no longer entice me to buy, but now serve to call attention to the many losses I've suffered.

Faced with these distractions, it's easy to lose oneself in the noise. When healthy, although I had an intellectual understanding of the basic tenets of Eastern thought, I found them nearly impossible to put into practice. Now that I'm sick, I find it just as impossible to not rely heavily upon them.

The literal translation of "the Tao" is "the Way", the inner path one must travel to find true happiness and contentment. This path can't be defined by outside influences, and is unique to each individual.

In fact, the wisdom contained within cannot be conveyed to you by anybody else, and in that way the Tao, your Tao, is unknowable to all but you. Only by quieting our inner turmoil, and turning down the cacophony of conflicting thoughts, emotions and desires, can we come to an understanding of our own personal path to fulfillment. We carry within us all that we need to be happy despite the chaos ricocheting around us, and if we can only learn to listen to these inner whispers we can undertake the necessary steps to create our own contented reality.

We are taught very early on that taking action, almost any action, should always be the goal, and the heroes in our society are always those whose actions speak the loudest. But the deeper truth is that sometimes more can be accomplished by inaction rather than action, an idea that might seem incongruous, at first glance.

The flow of life can be likened to a raging river, and too many of us spend our lives constantly trying to swim upstream, valiantly but hopelessly fighting the natural flow of our own lives, sometimes to the point of drowning, in a desperate attempt to reach what we have been led to believe is material and personal "success". If time and effort is spent putting aside those frantic efforts, and we quiet down long enough to discern the true direction in which life wants to lead us, the wise come to understand that by simply floating on their backs and relinquishing the struggle, they will finally reach their destination, a truer more fulfilling destination, and thus avoid the misery, heartache and inevitable discontent born of the perpetual battle.

Many Taoist lessons are taught through parable, and my favorite of these was first related by the ancient Tao Master, Chuang-tzu:

"There was a man who disliked seeing his footprints and his shadow. He decided to escape from them, and began to run. But as he ran along, more footprints appeared, while his shadow easily kept up with him. Thinking he must be going too slowly, he ran faster and faster without stopping, until he finally collapsed from exhaustion and died.

What a fool.

If he had stood still, there would have been no footprints. If he had rested in the shade, his shadow would have disappeared."

I've been aware of this parable for at least two decades, and was always struck by the simplicity and profundity of its wisdom. Now, afflicted with MS, its message has taken on immense new dimensions. My footprints are now tire tracks, and when I see my shadow I'm somehow still always shocked to see that the silhouette I make is no longer that of the strapping 6 footer I once was, but instead is that of a man in a wheelchair. MS has erased my footprints, and forced me to sit at rest. This reality is inescapable no matter how frantic my efforts, and running away is quite literally no longer an option.

The way, then, is to find the contentment within that eclipses physical disability, and to make the infinite number of choices each and every day that allow for that contentment. I will never be happy about having multiple sclerosis, but I can be happy in spite of it. My efforts to combat the disease will never cease, but in the tradition of the ancient warrior, my efforts to battle the illness are best born from tranquility and quiet determination, and not from the turmoil of desperation.

In the end, when pondering the imponderable, we simply must learn to let it be.

Let it be.

–Marc Stecker

Marc Stecker, aka The Wheelchair Kamikaze, is a 51-year-old male, living in New York City with his lovely and wonderful wife Karen. Diagnosed with Primary Progressive Multiple Sclerosis in March of 2003. http://www.wheelchairkamikaze.com

Reprinted from www.wheelchairkamikazee.com with permission of the author.

New Beginnings Equal Happier Endings

I can't do what I need due to severe fatigue, and I can try to explain but I can't articulate, even if I could get the words right, there is a good chance not a soul would relate, and this is all caused by this invisible illness, MS. They look and they say, "But you look so great", but they don't understand how this unfeigned migraine won't dissipate, or how hard one has to concentrate in order to walk. The literal spills, the physical falls, MS, where shooting pain and throbbing become one in the same, every single day, no break, way too mundane… something has to give, because I realize, I only have one life to live, and I still have the inner strength of a Mighty Hawk. First, I have to fix my fatigue, so in the process, my appetite, I will intrigue, with fresh fruits and vegetables and organic meats. And in the same way, faithfully, take my DMT's, so all of that insane pain, and all that throbbing that used to cause sobbing can go away. My days are now Blessed and no longer gray; I am alive and well with Multiple Sclerosis, what more can I say!

–Ashli Hopson

The Dreamer

The world we live in is an interesting place,
I wish everyone was able to have a smile on their face,
but because of certain life circumstances, unfortunately that isn't the case.
I wish more people asked me for hugs, and not requested me to leave and their space!

I wish we lived in a world where everyone was nice to each other,
one in which we didn't think twice before helping our sister or brothers.
I wish all doctors were outwardly fuzzy and warm like our mothers!

I wish we didn't laugh and mock at the things we don't understand,
I wish all wheelchairs went the speed of Dodge Caravans!
I wish everyone was patient and loving with their fellow man.

I wish bad things never happened to good human beings,
I wish when people spoke there were never double meanings.
I wish all the dogs that aided sick people were actually human beings!

I wish disease didn't have a place in our society,
I wish as opposed to one cure for each disease, there were more like ninety!

I wish getting a spinal tap was something no one had to dread,
I wish every single sick person was able to afford their med,
which would help combat these ailments, and man from being confined to their bed!

I wish Autoimmune disorders didn't exist,
I wish getting an MRI was all the rage and made you full of bliss!
I wish staying healthy was number one on everyone's list.

I wish MS didn't hurt so many so bad,
I wish nothing in this world could cause sorrow and everything made you glad.

–Ashli Hopson

The Survivor's Anthem

Keep hope alive; keep that willingness to thrive, yes, you are going to have to fight in order to survive. Now that we are here, a life with any less effort I cannot contrive. Keep hope alive; no, it does not mean your life is any less live, no need to feel deprived, but to the contrary, the opportunity is now and now we must dive, into our future knowing a cure is on the way, and I've used that very revelation as fuel for my drive, and as the basis for me to NEVER give up on my life.

–Ashli Hopson

Ashli Hopson was diagnosed with MS in 2007. In 2014, she was selected to be an MSF Ambassador. Currently, she is a Lead Patient Advisor for a MS research project. Her book *Sick, Not Stupid* is a memoir examining her past and present life with MS.

Solace

Edges
of brick
turning
shoes
into
toe
picks

Cane
symbol
look
sneer
words
of hope
silent

Touch
numb
lost
feet
ground
rumble
tumble

Breath
stabbing
hugs
crush
loved
one
not

Fear
hope
sleep
dream
no
more

solace

–Lisa Emrich

The Mermaid in the Pool

Once upon a time, many moons ago, there was a young mermaid. She lived on the land among the humans, yet did not know she was a mermaid.

In her dreams, she shared the ocean waters with the giant manatee and the baby sea turtles. When life on land became troublesome, she felt trapped in a riptide and dragged beneath the darkness. But when life was fine, the water was crystal clear against a blue sky.

The mermaid told of her dreams to a very good friend who suggested that she test the waters and go for a swim.

The water felt cool and the pressure against her limbs was soothing.

Swish, swish. The flowing, liquid bed rushing by her ears opened her soul to the Music of the Spheres.

A few trips to the pool and the mermaid was hooked. This was home.

She began to record each lap as she flew through the liquid air from pool edge to pool edge — each Monday, Wednesday, Friday — increasing the number of passes from day to day and week to week.

The mermaid thrilled at the very first time she swam a full mile in the pool. She had never swum this way before. Oh sure, she had splashed around in her younger years, but never relished in the flow of each backstroke.

Not before long, the mermaid saw clear blue skies and cool water during the day, every day, even while on land. The dark riptides had receded beyond the horizon.

The mermaid found herself smiling more often, carefree and light as a feather.

One day, as the mermaid was swimming glorious laps in the pool, flying through the water on the wings of swim flippers and stretching far overhead with each backstroke.... Wham!

Suddenly the mermaid hit a wall. Not the edge of the pool, but something nearly as hard and dangerous.

The mermaid had run head-on into a woman who had entered her lane and was lolly-gagging while chatting with friends.

Bam!! Right into the woman's back, the mermaid's flight came to a sudden halt.

"Damn, that hurt!!"

My head crashed straight down into my spine. Muscles tensed, headache surged, while my neck immediately felt "cricked."

The pain in my neck continued for days as I hoped to recover. My shoulders were tight and playing my french horn became uncomfortable. But discomfort is not unfamiliar to musicians who often play through various pains of which the audience is never aware.

The mermaid had a doctor's appointment just a few weeks after the crash in the pool and mentioned tingling in her left hand to her doctor. She and her doctor suspected a pinched nerve to be the cause of her pain and discomfort.

"Keep an eye on it and if it gets worse, let me know," said the doctor.

A month later my new Sweetie, whom I had recently just met, was gently rubbing my shoulders. Then he brushed my back.

"That's really weird. What's going on?" she thought.

The mermaid couldn't feel his hands on the left side of her back. The right side was fine, but the left side was numb.

Really numb.

So she called her doctor and scheduled a visit. Her left arm had become numb and tingly from fingertips to spine. Totally numb.

"I want you to have an MRI... just to get a better look at what might be going on in your neck," the doctor said.

The first trip through the MRI machine — the loudest, clang-y-est knock knock knock that ever hit human ears - showed spots. All in the neck, but spots nonetheless.

100 miles in the pool, a new neurologist, repeat MRIs, concerts in the park, spinal tap, veins flooded with solumedrol. This is the way the mermaid began her journey to a new life of living with multiple sclerosis.

I dreamt. I cried. And as tears mixed with chlorine, the mermaid became stronger and better able to face new realities on land.

Being diagnosed with MS is a life-changing event. Finding solace in the comfort of swimming laps in a warm pool can also be life-changing.

Through the challenges of MS, it is important to honor your 'mermaid' within. Continue to focus on who you are deep down and you will be able to find your way.

Take each day, one at a time. Each lap in the pool, one backstroke at a time. Each relapse, each challenge, each victory, one at a time.

–Lisa Emrich

Lisa Emrich, MM, teaches horn and piano and writes for several health-related websites. She was diagnosed with MS in 2005, five years after her first attack of optic neuritis, and with RA in 2007. Author of the award-winning blog, Brass and Ivory: Life with MS and RA, Emrich advocates for patient education, research, and self-empowerment.

Every Step I Take

Did you ever feel noticed? As a fourteen-year-old tenth grader, I moved fifteen miles with my family from Elmo's West Nodaway R-I school to North Nodaway R-I school in Hopkins. Leaving friends gathered from first grade on, I was suddenly new. During that first year, as some of the newness wore off, there were some teachers I liked and I began a part time job after school and weekends at Barnett's Hy-Klas grocery. Basketball, later so important, was just there. I was young and not grown up yet, but my sisters were in the middle school and they talked often about their coach Marvin Murphy.

Coach Murphy came to my high school when I was a junior. Early in the year he asked if I would be interested in being 'student trainer' for the football team. Liking the job description, I began to keep the team's statistics and filed its scorebooks with the stats after each game. During practices I did errands for the coaches.

Coach Murphy's own chiropractic training had stopped when he was drafted during WWII. After the war, he began professional life in coaching, teaching and educational administration. He shared his knowledge of muscle and bone structure, teaching me to give football players muscle rubdowns – on their shoulders, necks, backs, and calves. That was something I did every day as part of regular training during football season.

Basketball, though, was my main sport. In my senior high school year Coach made me a starting forward on the Varsity team. I was doing okay but one night I scored 30 points. After the game, in a room surrounded by teammates I was quietly getting dressed by my locker. My feelings were mixed: proud, disbelieving, practically overwhelmed. Coach Murphy usually went around the locker room after games. On this night as he came by I said I couldn't believe it. He put his arm around me saying, "I knew you could do it, and you'll do it again!" Over and over I did.

One night we played Forrest City. They had a star player, Dennis Klassmeyer, who routinely scored 30-40 points a game, a lot for a high school player. Forrest City's season team record was better than that of my North Nodaway. Before the game, Coach told the rest of our team he wanted me to abandon our traditional zone defense, because wanted me to go one on one with Denny Klassmeyer.

"Be in his face all the time," Coach Murphy said to me, "and don't let up. When he doesn't have the ball, be between him and the ball, uptight in front of him!" After the game, Coach came by player lockers as he always did. When he was by me I said to him, "Klassmeyer is all-star material!" "Yes he is," responded Coach, "but you held him to 7 points."

During those three final years of high school, in addition to being student manager for the football team, playing track and basketball I took driver's education from Coach Murphy and a mandatory heath class, but I have several further memories of him.

First, one Saturday morning after my senior basketball season, Coach Murphy met me in the gym where he had played for his college Alma Mater. He had arranged an introduction to Dick Buckridge the college basketball coach. When fall came I did try out for the college team, but Coach Buckridge told Coach Murphy that three new freshmen had made the team. I was the fourth, but the cafeteria of college life had already become exciting. Basketball was important, but there seemed so much to sample, learn and do.

Years later I was a new teacher in an old boys school in New York City. Two years prior to my employment they had admitted girls for the first time, and they wanted a basketball team. The coaching staff was already fully committed but my previous experience in basketball was known and I was asked to be the girls coach. Of course I was willing, but you might guess who my model was as we won a few games with some wonderful girls.

When my Missouri high school graduation's fortieth reunion arrived, I had lived for years in New York City, but I went back to see classmates. Coach Murphy came to the reunion in full coach's regalia, including baseball cap. Retired by then, he was solely devoted to his adult sport of softball. Always interested in girl's athletics, he had become Missouri's foremost girls' softball pitching coach.

Coach had been a summertime softball pitcher when I had known him during high school, and I had memories of catching for him each spring as he conditioned his arm for the summer season. Fond memories might be an inaccurate description, as his pitches were amazingly fast and hard. While I could catch them, to this non-softball player my glove seemed thin as paper. At the fortieth reunion, he and I had our picture taken together. That photo of him and me, with his ever-present coach's baseball cap, will always be part of my photo archives.

In 2008 Mom sent me Coach Murphy's obituary from a local Maryville paper, the Daily Forum. A funny man, Coach had always called that paper the Daily Fool – em. Though his corporeal presence has left this earth, I still think of him daily. I realize how important he was to my 'physical' education and sense of self in this world. He sought me out, offering steady encouragement. When I was proud he applauded, but I often realize that in true coaches fashion he had seen it there before it ever happened.

Coach Murphy always said, "Girls don't know how to punch!" That didn't stop him from teaching them in every girls gym class each year. As I help lead punching exercises in my assisted living now I laugh, as those older women punch straight ahead, straight up, round houses, and finally finish off with upper cuts. I tell them, "If only Coach Murphy could see us now!"

Pursuing my goal to be a walking guy after thirteen years of going the opposite direction, Coach Murphy's voice is for sure inside my head. As I walk now, I think of how I learned to stand and move in balance as an athlete under his guidance. Somewhere I learned the term 'kinesthetic awareness' and I don't know if that term came from Coach or not. Certainly it was what he always talked about, being aware of where you were, how you were doing it, and what might come next. As I walk with the formerly broken right leg from a fall, that doesn't fit quite like I remember from when I used to walk, I think every step I take of how Coach might say to do it right.

–Ronald Huff

Ronald Huff was born in Missouri, leaving at twenty-four for graduate school in New York City at Union Seminary. Twenty years later, he had spent his early adulthood there as an educator. Disabled at forty-four by MS, he has spent time since writing and doing various volunteer work.

This Wretched MS and Me

Got a tremor in my hand
Call it my "Shaky Shit,"
Had to get home health-care
To help me deal with it.

It's spreading thru my body
Looks like Parkinson's Disease,
Feel like Katherine Hepburn
Really Karma? Please.

Look drunk while walking
As I ricochet off walls,
Maintaining my dignity
Really takes some balls.

My balance is shot
Bladder is weak,
Have to wear Depends
In case I spring a leak.

When my RLS flares up
My knees jerk wildly,
I laugh & shrug it off
This wretched MS and me.

–Angela Allen

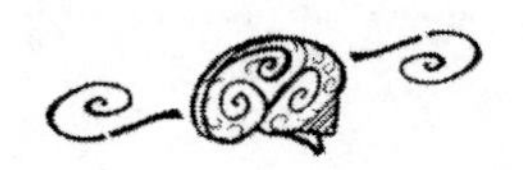

I Can Still ...

I can still BREATHE on my own
And it's good.

I can still BATHE, FEED, and DRESS myself
And it's gratifying.

I can still SEE the sky
And it's beautiful.

I can still HEAR the thunder
And it's awesome,

I can still FEEL the wind
And it's refreshing.

I can still THINK for myself
And it's satisfying.

I can still HELP people
And it's rewarding.

I can still ENCOURAGE others
And it's fulfilling.

I can still DO a lot of things for myself
And I'm GRATEFUL.

–Angela Allen

The Wheelchair Cruise

I can't drive a car
Or walk very far,
But I don't lose I take
A wheelchair cruise.

When I roll down the road
People tend to stare,
But it ain't no biggie
Coz I just don't care.

It is what it is
It ain't what it ain't,
I'll do what I can do
And I won't what I cain't.
There are certain times
When I get the blues,
But when that happens
I do the wheelchair cruise.

She can outrun dogs that
Chase me down the street,
There ain't nothin' this
Ole' chair cain't beat.

She has four speeds
Toppin' 15 mile an hour,

Has quite a rev' and is
Chalk full of power.

That's the reason why
I can put on my shoes,
And with no shame I
Do the wheelchair cruise.

–Angela Allen

I Went to the Doctor

I went to the Doctor...
another check-up,
Soon be on my way
After peein' in a cup.

When they got the results
I was rolled down the hall,
Told to wait right there
And my name they'd call.

I twiddled my thumbs
Tried to read a book,
I couldn't concentrate
So all I did was look.

Right across the way
An elderly fellow sat,
He was sawin' logs
'Neath a big straw hat.

On the rug over there
Sat two small boys,
Havin' a battle
Squablin' over toys.

Mama hovered near
Gabbin' on the phone,
Her sister was in town
And all alone.

The chair in the corner
Held a pretty little girl,
In a flowery dress
With hair all a-curl.

A teen entered the room
Long hair over eyes,
Actin' so cool,
Lookin' so wise

.

The air was very cold
It was 90' outside,
All I could think of
Was a long Harley ride.

Startled out of sleep when
My name they did call.
I grabbed my cane
Stumbled down the hall.

The nurse took my vitals
Put me on the scale,
She took my temperature
Asked if I felt well.

Before I knew it
I was layin' on a gurney
Racin' thru the halls on
An unexpected journey.

The last I remember
Was an oxygen mask,
Falling from above
Intent on its task.

Two days later
I was home again.
With a groggy head and
No memory where I'd been.

–Angela Allen

Angela D. Morgan Allen was diagnosed with RRMS in July of 2003. An amateur writer, photographer, and digital artist, she uses her talents to advocate for MS and disabilities in general. Her poems are a combination of encouragement, truth, questions, frustration, humor and attitude relating to the difficulties of living with MS.

Finding Joy Amongst Pain

Therapy comes in many forms. Writing is my therapy in dealing with a chronic illness that is constantly getting worse. Faith in God, courage to confront this daily degeneration of my nervous system, and reflection has led me on a journey I hope others can benefit from. But prayer is my salvation. Scripture helps me daily and favorites are shared within.

On October 11, 2010, the diagnosis of Multiple Sclerosis was given to me over the phone by a neurologist. I had my second MRI a week before. What kind of doctor gives out a prognosis over the phone, I thought. "Come into my office and we'll talk," he said. He described the diagnosis and its meaning for over an hour and took all of my questions. I finally had a name to call my maladies. At least it's not cancer, I told him. Only if I'd have known. Most cancer can be treated and cured. **Primary Progressive Multiple Sclerosis (PPMS)** cannot. Over the course of the next few days, I investigated this illness at the library and online. Symptoms I had previously experienced began making sense. On my own I began to figure out what all of this information meant. My partner had earlier questioned me over the thought of multiple sclerosis after researching my symptoms of imbalance, falling, afternoon fatigue and walking with a limp. I had brushed her off one or two days previous. Now I had to deal with the idea of MS.

Imagine falling headfirst in slow motion. You know you're headed down but you can't stop it. Thoughts of what to do pass through your mind but you just wait to hit the sidewalk. Should my hand go first or my arm? What will hurt most? Imagine... suddenly tripping over your feet for no apparent reason. Nothing was found to help me understand what my body was going through with walking difficulties. I turned to prayer and affirmations.

Trust in the Lord with all your heart, and do not lean on your own understanding.
In all your ways acknowledge him,
and he will make straight your paths. (Proverbs 3:5-6)

Another scenario: slowly over months your fingers/ hands/ toes tingle like there's no blood in your veins. How about feeling exhausted all day long for no reason; what would you do?

Most books and pamphlets acknowledge PPMS but seldom inform us on therapies and treatment. I learned on my own most chiropractors or physical therapists don't know or understand the forms of MS and how to help those with special needs. Once I began researching MS I noticed how little focus was placed on progressive types. I dug deeper into websites targeting neurological illnesses. A cane arrived in the mail but I chose to ignore it for over a year: I wasn't prepared to need a mobility device just then.

Dear God,
Today I woke up. I'm alive. I'm blessed.
I apologize for all my complaining.
I'm truly grateful for all you have done in my life.

Three years after diagnosis I had to retire from teaching. I began reading from Buddhist practitioners on mindfulness, breathing practices and meditation. I read from several reference sources how meditation reduces stress, helps repair ill health and gives you energy and I began appreciating little joys in my life. I have much to feel blessed for and continue to realize these gifts. Simple things like sharing new information on what works for me fighting symptoms or learning new tricks to deal with limitations makes me feel purposeful.

Humble yourselves, therefore, under the mighty
hand of God so that at the proper time
He may exalt you, casting all your anxieties on him,
because He cares for you. (1 Peter 5:6-7)

My first weapon against MS became juicing; 'drinking' organic vegetables and fruits for their phytonutrients, within ten minutes of juicing. I experienced an increase in energy by consuming large amounts of greens was a benefit within days. I use mostly kale, spinach, celery, apples, cucumbers and parsley. But I found recipes for other drinks requiring beets and carrots, pears, chard, broccoli, cilantro and cactus. Functional Nutrition has been coined recently to encompass eating specific foods to achieve optimum health.

It's easy for me to try something new when progression brings about worsening movement and pain. Reading and witnessing YouTube videos about symptom control through specific food diets and functional medicine are highly hopeful, especially if it makes logical sense. Food should be healthy: whole, non-GMO (genetically-modified organisms), organic, nutritious. We eat as healthy as possible every day of our lives. I read other sources and began improving my diet. Now I find an increase in studies and articles that support and promote diets for increased energy, vitality and clarity. If it's not going to help, why eat it.

"Let food be thy medicine and medicine be thy food." Hippocrates

Fighting fatigue is a daily struggle for people with MS. This fatigue is not your typical tiredness due to low energy or overexertion. For me, it encompasses heaviness throughout my body weighing me down while feeling exhaustion with every step or breath. I often find myself with so little energy and I can become lost in thought no matter where I am, be it the toilet, bed, couch or kitchen chair. I can't work anymore; the need for speed is a thing of the past. When I move it means feeling pain, but it didn't always. The strange feeling of heaviness in my lower body kept me dragging as I walked: moving in slow motion.

In the first month of diagnosis I realized the importance of keeping a journal on *my* therapy routine and symptom management. I was losing confidence in the medical profession. My doctor said there were no other drugs or therapies for me. My new disabled placard was ordered. Movement is slow and difficult; my left foot usually getting in the way with my toes turned over, my shoe scraping the ground.

The first walking aid I used was an AFO, a foot orthotic molded of plastic in an L-shape to keep the toes from turning under, causing trips and falls. The new brace was a Godsend. I was mobile again, until I needed a cane. I could walk and my brace was hidden under my slacks.

I first blamed this severe tiredness on menopause. Energy came with a daily brew of roots from my acupuncturist. To keep up the added energy, I sought other methods from many sources, not understanding the cause of the fatigue. While working, I found myself explaining to coworkers that I'm not lazy or non-productive, but without education of this chronic illness, society sees us as healthy individuals. We don't look sick; canes and walkers give away our need for mobility needs but the corrosion of our nervous system is hidden away. We want to scream, "Hey, I'm not drunk!" when we show balancing problems. I couldn't raise my arm or use my hand due to loss of dexterity and strength. Although there is strength in my hands, I can no longer use my right one.

Getting ready in the morning can take a long time and wear me out. Learning that others experience the same by listening in MS Support Groups makes me feel normal in my new community. My new normal includes a cold, numb right hand and foot, the need to sit after getting dressed, take naps, and procrastination. Without my partner, who is also my caregiver, to help me with my hair, some clothing and cooking 80% of meals, I wouldn't make it. Preparing a meal is a major endeavor.

I'm not alone in my struggle. My partner of several years has been there for me long before I received my diagnosis. She helped me up when I fell, diagnosed me using the Internet, supported me through every challenge and never gave up loving. I never thought about the effort and patience a caregiver requires until my father's aggressive dementia took its toll on my mother. Caregivers need a 'caregiver' for them, too — caregivers can burn out. They need to care for themselves at the same time and always be alert. We are fortunate to have a caregivers' support group. There the caregivers can gather information, tips on coping and sharing of experiences; the support of others and professionals can be of utmost importance.

Spasticity and Pain

Neurologists, unless they have MS,
Don't know what it's like
To wake up to extreme, pulsating leg pain
Minutes after standing,
Bending for relief,
Groaning to stem the razor sharp stings
In your thighs and legs.
Hold on to the counter!
Brace yourself!
It's like muscles somersaulting
While burning sensations under your skin
shoot through every nerve ending.
Why isn't the muscle relaxant working?
I silently pray while standing,
Waiting for the pain to subside.

II

My leg, stiffened.
Walking forward is difficult.
My foot drags clumsily.
I can't pick up my leg and move it ahead.
I stop suddenly and rest to proceed again.
Walking forward is difficult.
If I swing out my useless leg,
I can move faster.

It just won't bend on its own.

I'm tired.

Walking forward is difficult.

III

Laying down

A sharp pain through my right thigh

Jerks my leg up just as I'm about to doze.

My leg feels cold, hard.

I try to move over; but

My body doesn't budge.

Upright

Bending over

Hurts.

My trunk is stone-like, dead weight.

I rub my thigh for warmth

But that doesn't work.

Eventually my legs relax

After spasms or

Until I move again.

The MS muscle relaxant Baclofen can take away some of my muscle tightening sensations and pain. Many drugs leave you with a side effect, this one is sleepiness. I've since doubled the dosage but after a month, I feel no lessening of heaviness in my legs and back, tightness while moving or sitting. What will happen when I reach the highest dosage allowed and still no relief? Movement of a body that feels like stone but looks healthy and 'normal' is a permanent trial. I change the dosage and times I take the white pills. Feels like such a 'crap shoot' with trial by error. I'm a guinea pig. My life is all about relieving the pain, which didn't exist with the spasticity two years earlier.

MS spasms arrive daily like pain only they last for seconds producing leg jerks and jumps, usually when I first lay down or sit down. Spasms sneak up at night or in the morning. These sudden jerks slowly subside. Four years after diagnosis, I began experiencing what's known as 'the MS hug', tightness around the abdomen that sporadically comes and goes. The heaviness I experienced before losing the 'gluten gut' reappeared. It's as if I'm wearing a corset and someone pulls it taunt at whim.

Typical of MS fatigue, unlike being exhausted, the sufferer doesn't feel refreshed after a ten-hour sleep. You long to stay in the bed. Pulling yourself out involves energy, stamina and balance, all at the same time. Some days I don't feel like doing anything, which includes dressing. It is such a laborious task. My legs feel heavy and huge, yet I'm a size 10, 138 lb. frame at 5'6''. With MS, neurons in the cells in my brain and spinal cord can't make the connections. Degeneration has left these neurons floating around looking for someone to hook-up with, or so I visualize it to understand. I feel like I'm dragging cement weights on my legs and feet, around my abdomen. A few steps taken anywhere make me tired. Once I'm seated, I don't want to arise from the chair, unless, of course, pain in my thighs touching the chair causes me to move. These burning sensations subside with time. My thoughts linger to a sleep state, but I'm not sleepy, just tired. Moving my legs takes more energy than ever before. Before diagnoses, when massage therapists would ask me to turn over so they could massage my back, it felt difficult and strange. My body felt weighted down and three or four times as heavy as my entire weight. It was another sign something was wrong.

Muscle weakness presented itself when I couldn't lift my right arm to write on the board in my classroom, pull myself up on a chair to create a bulletin board, or move to music in a salsa dance. To my surprise, both of my neurologists have tested my arm strength and confirmed my arms to be as strong as before, my brain no longer makes the connection to what my body has and what it can do. I use a stationary bike and a vibration machine daily for exercise. But some days I take a break; I'm just too exhausted.

MS fatigue involves muscle fatigue, brain or cognitive fatigue and physical fatigue all at once. Cognitive fatigue is a clear sign it is time to stop working. Students in my classes tried to finish my sentences. Words failed me. Phrases couldn't come together. As an English teacher, this was unacceptable. I began to forget simple things at home and let pots burn, the kitchen timer melt, unpaid bills were forgotten. The end result brought on laughter for the moment, but continuous brain fog got the best of me. Looking back, the sense of clouded thought was about five times what I experienced from menopause.

MS Support Groups have helped in understanding specific concerns like cognition, mood and fatigue. We share concerns around the table and offer advice, wisdom or information. Each session brings a new understanding about minor experiences that make a major difference in how I understand my situation. Sometimes just knowing you're not alone makes the group such an invaluable tool for getting through another two weeks. Family participation in yearly MS Walks rejuvenates me and gives me strength.

"Come to me, all who labor and are heavy laden, and I will give you rest. Take my yoke upon you, and learn from me, for I am gentle and lowly in heart, and you will find rest for your souls. For my yoke is easy, and my burden is light."

(Matthew 11:28-30)

Brain games hopefully push my cognitive skills. I eat for improved brain health. So many of my troubles seem to be associated with my brain: thinking, making connections, memory, mood, and speech. Lucky for me, brain games have recently gained attention and are quite helpful in fighting atrophy of brain muscles.

Now my pain coincides with my spasticity in my legs and various spasms or under-the-skin burning sensations of my thighs. Some responds to medicinal cannabis (CBD pills, rub, edibles). A warm bath with Epsom salts and hot jets in a whirlpool feel good during the time of the soak only.

Dr. Rosalind Kalb refers to places, physically or mentally, where one can forget for a while that they have MS. Or it could slip the mind because you are enjoying life's many joys and your diagnoses moves to the background. Now I find it so necessary. Therapeutic warm pool stretches and exercises give me relief until I get out. Soaking in a whirlpool has always given me great pleasure until I get out. It's all about looking for pleasure amongst pain, relief no matter how long. Diet, physical and mental exercise, connection to others through support groups online and in community all provide me with a sense of hope through my journey. Through sharing my experience, I hope for a better understanding of our plight by medical professionals and caregivers of chronic illnesses.

–Constance Chevalier

Constance Chevalier is a former middle school and high school Language Arts teacher, mother of two grown children, and avid reader. With an interest and ability in photography, she traveled to Cuba, Costa Rica, Nicaragua and Italy before it became too problematic.

Rome Wasn't Built In a Day . . .

You Can't Storm the Appian Way

Dr. Greenstein gave me a thorough check-up. That included tuning fork hearing tests, flashlights for my eyes to follow side to side then up and down, sharp objects touching each hand and foot while my eyes were closed, a hands-on strength test all over both arms and legs, a look at my latest MRI on a 3×3 screen, a walk across the room holding him on one side and my son on the other. We all sat down again. His written file on me at the nearby table was 1 ½ inches thick.

He looked at me (the new owner of a third electric wheelchair) and said, "I want you to walk again." He outlined his plan, and we discussed how he wanted to do it. He said his goal was for me to be able to use my crutches again. I was overwhelmed, that anyone would care so much. My emotions rolled from my eyes down my cheeks, as I said, "I had never expected to walk again!"

Giving a prescription for Ritalin (at its lowest dose) and one for Physical Therapy (PT) aimed specifically toward walking, he ended the visit saying, "I will see you in a month to evaluate." Three weeks later PT Charol measured me walking 225 feet with a walker, taking a rest, and walking back. In four visits Charol had taught me several new leg exercises and we began to run a gauntlet of increasing demands and difficulty. I found myself wondering if my three pairs of Lofstrand crutches were still stored at my son's house.

At the one-month follow up with Dr. Greenstein, the Ritalin dosage was increased to 10 mg, taken three times daily at mealtime. A prescription for Physical Therapy, just for walking, was renewed.

Tomorrow I see him again. Since my last visit my measured walking distance and my standing time have both more than doubled. I step sideways and backwards with the skill of a clumsy ballerina. The hallway outside my room has hosted a slalom course of paper cups to successfully navigate.

During Tuesday's Physical Therapy I left my room on a walker, continuing down the hallway to the elevator. Taking it downstairs to the living room I rested in a chair and then came back to my room and through the door. Friday, I went down the same elevator, this time continuing to the lunchroom. Sitting in a chair at my table

In the far end of that lunchroom I took a break. Then I retraced my steps and took the reverse elevator trip to my room. There are no negative side effects from Ritalin or from increased, new exercises.

PT Charol says we will do the Dining Room routine once more for practice, but after that I can do it alone. Tomorrow, I have another follow up with Dr. Greenstein. Hey, I used to say that a good day was being able to stand up and pull my pants up with two hands. Now, I'm beginning to think of myself as a stand-up kind of guy. No, Rome wasn't built in a day. And what I have described sometimes seemed like training for the Olympics — but look at me: having read this to a group as I stand before them.

–Ronald Huff

Ronald Huff was born in Missouri, leaving at twenty-four for graduate school in New York City at Union Seminary. Twenty years later, he had spent his early adulthood there as an educator. Disabled at forty-four by MS, he has spent time since writing and doing various volunteer work.

Dancing with Multiple Sclerosis

My name is Brieana Straiton, most people call me Brie. I live in Bloomington, Minnesota and work as a Customer Loyalty Rep for Comcast. After growing up in a small town, at the age of 16 my Mom moved us back to the city. I didn't stay there for long. A few weeks before my 18th birthday, I met my now husband, Ryan, working at Subway. He convinced me to move to California with him. We lasted out there for about 2 years before finances forced us to move back to MN. It was the best and the worst decision I'd made moving out there. So much drama. So many memories of the ocean and all the beautiful things California holds. I'd love to move back someday.

When I came back to MN it was May 2005. Ryan got a job the same day at a pizza place called Davanni's. I ended up getting a job there about a month later as a driver. We both worked there on and off, mostly on for me, for about 8 yrs. During that time, we went to college and attained AAS degrees. Ryan got lucky and was able to get a job in his field. I wasn't as lucky. At the time, I was only working 1 day a week at Davanni's and had a temp job drafting plumbing lines. I was sure I'd get hired but I didn't so it was back to Davanni's for me. We were married a few months later on Sept 7th, 2008. Life was great for a few years, but once that time was over, it was really over.

Fast forward to 2013 and enter from stage left, Multiple Sclerosis. I was diagnosed on Sept 29th 2013 with RRMS. This story is a true account of my life shortly before and after my diagnosis.

In order to really grasp my state of mind during this tumultuous time, it's important a few base facts are known. At the beginning of 2013 my husband, Ryan, and I were on the verge of divorce. I had cheated on Ryan. Since that's a story all its own, I'll leave that for my book to explain. The emotional turmoil and stress of that situation is what, I believe, caused my MS to rear its ugly head.

July in Minnesota: hot, humid, and sticky. For us city dwellers, a few hours drive north to a cabin or camping means cooler temps on average. It also leads to 'destination weddings'. My bestie of 19 years, Mary, choose to take advantage of this "backyard" beauty for her wedding. Her ceremony was held at the Grand View Lodge in Nisswa, MN out on Gull Lake. I was the Maid of Honor so there was no missing this for me.

A week before the wedding Ryan moved back in after almost 2 months of living with his Mom. He had not been invited to the wedding after an altercation with the Groom a few months before. Ryan wasn't OK with me being gone for 4 days to say the least. We fought constantly. It was so stressful, so sad. I was to leave Thursday morning. By Tuesday I woke up unable to focus my eyes. It was a cross between double and blurred vision. I couldn't even watch TV. Once I would wake up and get my contacts in it seemed to get a little better. The wedding was beautiful, from what I could see at least, but between the vision problem and Ryan's constant calls and texts, it felt like I wasn't there. The drive home on Sunday was about 5 hours due to traffic. By Monday my vision was back to normal. I was so caught up in my life I didn't give it a second thought.

A few weeks later I ended up at the doctor's office with a severe double ear infection. My left ear was far worse than the right. The doctor said the inside of my ear was the color of a tomato. Due to the level of infection and swelling he gladly gave me a few Percocet to get me through until the antibiotics kicked in.

Two days later I was called into work early. I got out of bed and into my uniform and out the door I went. When I got called in like that I would bring my contacts and makeup with me to work so I could be there ASAP. When I walked into the kitchen I was met by the confused and concerned faces of my co-workers. My boss asked me if I had looked in the mirror yet. I was like "Really? I just rolled out of bed and came here!" She suggested I take a look. I was shocked. I looked like I had had a stroke! The entire left side of my face was droopy. I had no control over my mouth or eyelids. My immediate reaction was panic. I called my doctor's office and they were able to squeeze me in later that afternoon. So I worked my shift and tried to stay focused. My mind raced the entire time. I did my best to keep cool.

By 1pm my nerves were completely frayed. When I got in my car, I broke down in tears. I looked in my rear view mirror and thought to myself, "This is it? This is how I will look for the rest of my life?" I drove the 10 miles from Eagan to Bloomington. I arrived at the clinic and checked in. Within a few minutes they whisked me back into one of the rooms. The nurse asked me the usual questions, allergies, current meds, etc. She took my vitals and told me to try to calm down and relax since my blood pressure and pulse were extremely high. Here I'm thinking to myself, "Are you fucking serious?? Fuckin right I'm stressed out!! I'm 28 and look like I've had a fucking stroke!"

Finally the doctor comes in. She tells me that she's my regular doctor's PA and she will figure out what's going on. I burst into tears and ask, "Did I have a stroke?" She assures me that no, I did not have a stroke. After a barrage of questions and some poking around on my face she announces, "You are suffering from Bell's Palsy. It looks like a stroke since it only affects 1 side of the face. The main nerve that controls those muscles runs very close to the ear canal. Since you have such a severe ear infection the inflammation caused the surrounding tissue to put pressure on that main nerve, thus slowing or stopping its function of muscle control on that side of your face." I must've looked confused. She grabbed one of her diagrams to explain it all further. She decided to add steroids to my mix and send me to an ENT (ear, nose, throat) doctor.

I was able to get in with the ENT doctor within a few days. He did a bunch of testing and looking inside of my ears before sending me off to have my hearing tested. The test took about 25 minutes. Then I sat and waited again. The doctor came in and explained that I had lost about 30% of the hearing in my left ear. As he was about to leave, I asked him, " What about this tingling numbness in my right leg? What explains that?" He turned and asked me to describe the sensation I was feeling in my upper right thigh. After a few more questions he said, "This is most likely a neurological problem so I'm going to refer you to a neurologist."

The referral was to the Minneapolis Clinic of Neurology in Burnsville. After 30 minutes on the phone with scheduling, they found an opening the next day with Dr. Evan Williams. As I walked into Suite 100 I was suddenly surrounded by old people in their walkers and wheelchairs accompanied by whatever poor sap from their family that had to deal with this. My anxiety takes over. I'm sweating and shaky and the room feels like is spinning and getting smaller. Just as I'm about to break, I see a tall young man in front of me. "Are you Brieana?" he says in a calming voice. "Yes" I answered meekly.

I followed him back to his office. He could see how apprehensive I was and proceeded to ask me to take a seat on the exam table. As he began the exam, I found myself looking around his office trying to ascertain how experienced he was, what his credentials were, and where he went to school. As he's poking around testing all my reflexes and strength I take a good, long look at him. He has an aura of sweetness that's very calming. This tall, lanky man who began balding way before his time now holds my fate. He confirms that the Bell's Palsy was most likely caused by the ear infection. His concern was my leg. Since there was nothing obvious from the outside, he ordered an MRI. I set the appointment with his nurse, Maureen, and was on my way out with more questions than answers.

Ryan's Dad had just invited us up north with them for the weekend to help us get some time together and try to heal the wounds between us. I was excited to go back to the North Shores of Lake Superior. I hadn't been since I was a child. We were able to get the MRI scheduled before we were set to leave. It was outside of the Minneapolis Clinic of Neurology clinics since none of them had openings. Instead they were able to get me in at Suburban Imaging in Edina.

I'd never been inside an MRI before, only a CT. This was very different. I walked in with Ryan, palms sweaty and heart racing. Once I found the correct office, I checked in and sat. My MRI tech was a young man who looked exhausted from the busy day but was still very patient and sweet. He told me to change into one of their gowns and make sure there was no metal left on my body. When I was done, he lead me into a room with this giant machine and told me to lay on the platform.

He explained how the machine worked and what to expect then proceeded to lock me in. They provided headphones for me to listen to local radio. I chose the oldies station hoping some Zeppelin or Journey would come on to relax me. The MRI…is…so…loud. I could barely hear the music. The confinement and noise made me claustrophobic. I kept my eyes shut the whole time. In about 35 minutes the scan was finished and the young tech came back into the room, pulled me out of the MRI, and removed the harness. I felt so relieved. That moment of relief and bliss was just that; a moment. My mind raced. "What will they see? Maybe I don't have MS so then what? Back to the drawing board? I want to know what the hell is wrong with me!" Once I found my way back to the waiting room after traversing what felt like a labyrinth to get there, I clung to Ryan and we walked back to our car. Even through all the drama I was so glad he was there with me.

Once back in the car, Ryan calmed me down and we were back on the road to the North Shores. Ryan put on some of my favorite music and tried his best to alleviate my fears. It was dusk when we arrived at the campsite. We stopped by to say hi to his dad and his wife at their site and out where we were supposed to set up. Ryan and I went to set up our site and change since it gets pretty cold on the shores at night, even in August. We spent about a week up there. The awe and beauty of nature has always had a calming effect on me so by the time we got back I was feeling better… though I still looked like I had had a stroke.

I saw Dr. Williams a few days later to review the results of the MRI. He found questionable spots, but wasn't quite convinced it was MS. Next step to determine if this is truly MS, a lumbar puncture, aka the spinal tap. As soon as the words left his mouth I was consumed by fear and anxiety. He assured me this was the best way to determine my diagnosis. I reluctantly went to Maureen to schedule the LP. She saw the apprehension on my face and attempted to calm my fears. We made the appointment for a few days later and then I went home.

The LP took place at Fairview Ridges Hospital. It felt like I was going in for surgery or something. I got all prepped and began to cry. "This could change my life forever." It was a painful experience. I left the hospital with lower back pain and many doubts running through my mind. They told me the results would take a few weeks.

Over the next few weeks my life went from sad to complete train wreck. My little brother Taylor destroyed his aortic valve by using dirty needles. He'd been a heroin addict for years and now it was killing him. He needed the valve replaced ASAP so open heart surgery was scheduled. On top of all this, my Grandpa had a heart attack. He turned out to be fine, but still, more stress and emotional discord for me. Taylor stayed in the hospital for the week prior to the surgery, so I spent a lot of my free time there. All this started to affect my ability to work and my performance began to slip.

After almost 10 years working at Davanni's I was fired for "incompetence." My boss had already mentioned she thought that I had MS. They all knew the official diagnosis was coming soon which meant that the ADA would have my back. I was blind-sided. I sat down in front of my 2 managers and our District Manager and was accused of being inappropriate and immature and told that there was no longer a place for me there. It was devastating. After so long the crew were my friends, my family, my little kids. It hurt my heart not being able to be around them more than losing job itself. I threw my hat, keys and access card on the counter and sobbing I said, "Thank you for ruining my life. Hope you're happy with that."

So to sum up: Taylor's life threatening surgery. Fired from my long time job. Ryan and I were back at each other's throats and he moved to his dad's house. I lost my apartment and had 6 days to move out. And the cherry on top? An official diagnosis of MS. The levels of distress, depression, self-pity, anger, sadness, fatigue and the feeling of my heart breaking was too much to bear. I spent '6 days in hell' trying to move all our stuff out of our home of 5 years into an 8x11 storage locker. Even thinking about now makes my heart ache.

After the '6 days in hell' I lived out of my car and slept wherever there was room. I rotated between my bestie's house, my mom's, Ryan's dad's place and my car. It was a depressing few weeks before Ryan and I decided to try again. His dad was nice enough to let us stay until we got back on our feet. It was a very difficult 10 months. I spent most of it locked away in our tiny room with my cat watching Netflix and dwelling in my own spiral of self-pity. After trying Copaxone and Tecfidera, with no improvement whatsoever, Dr. Williams decided to send me to the specialist he'd been consulting with about my case, Dr. Jonathan Calkwood of the Schapiro Center for Multiple Sclerosis. I've been under his care ever since. Since that time my life has changed so much. I have a great job with Comcast and they have been wonderful dealing with me and my MS. I've been on paid short-term disability since March 2015, but they never forget about me. Ryan and I are stronger than ever and are back to living on our own. We even got another cat, Skittles. My MS is still hitting hard. And I am learning to cope. I'm currently on Tysabri. Some of my lesions are shrinking. It's the symptoms that are killing me now. I have a hard time walking, hearing loss, major fatigue, and innumerable types of pain. I could go on...

Adapting has been hard on both of us, but Ryan has been there. I look at it as a death of sorts of my old self. That part of me is gone most likely forever. I accept that. But there is new life after an "MS Death." I've had to rebuild so many aspects of my life that

I am not who I once was. I've found a new happiness and purpose in life. For a long time after my diagnosis I considered my life over, but now almost 2 years later I see beyond the self-pity. What I see ahead looks brighter than ever even with the unknowns that come with having MS.

–Brieana Straiton

Brieana Straiton, aka Brie, lives in Bloomington, Minnesota, a suburb of Minneapolis. She is 30 years old and married to a wonderful man, Ryan. In September 2013 she was diagnosed with RRMS. She is very grateful for her loving family and friends who've been so supportive.

Invocation *to Beauty*

Oh!—whatever, Beauty! You drive a hard
    bargain: you'll toy with my shrinking good
looks only so much, and I will allow you to pilfer
    my expensive wardrobe for all the things
my crippled body can no longer wear: high-heeled
    shoes, their rhinestone toes swinging from
your exquisitely manicured hands—next, my dresses—
    slits on sheer crepe, short swingy skirts,
and blushing strapless beauties. But you went too far,
    dear Beauty—you clutch (tightly, I might add),
my tender cashmere sweaters to your wondrous bosom,
    your pink mouth puckering for a kiss,
your Victoria's Secret eyes lowered to softly rouged
    cheeks—and weren't you prancing on *Dancing
with the Stars*, twirling in my high heels while caressing
    the sable wrap that I didn't know you had stolen?
Although when I couldn't find it on the closet's top
    shelf where I keep precious things, I gave you
the benefit of the doubt, Beauty, you vixen, believing
    that you wouldn't betray me since we had
announced a truce: I would not expose your treachery
    and you would allow me to walk and keep

my smile—but your hesitancy in shaking my hand

to seal the deal told the tale of betrayal,

dear Beauty (the knife stab wounds to this day).

I have not been the same since you, Beauty,

with all your glitz and glamour, sat demurely in the back

seat, my sapphire and diamond necklace flashing

at the nape of your soft neck, while the Burden of disability

sat up front with me, and madly drove the car.

–Marie Kane

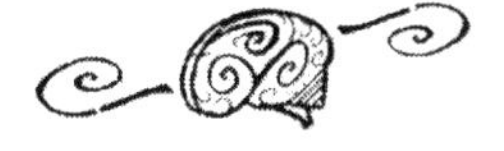

This Is the Life

So what if gods, fates, genetic
mysteries haven't been kind?
We all have our crosses and I don't
believe in the ecumenical notion
that all crosses are equal so no cosmic deal
with God would allow me
to place someone else here.
Hell, *I* don't want to be here.

Lying on the bedroom floor after falling, thirty
minutes pass while I straighten
my spastic legs, roll over on my stomach, hunch
knees and carbon fiber leg brace
under my chest, use my husband's dresser to pull
myself upright, praying it doesn't topple.

Sudden realization—practice acceptance—agree,
concur, assent, swallow whole.
And what if instead I choose refusal, opposition,
disagreement, rejection?
Now, here are the important questions: Why didn't I
revere running when I could? Adore
pain in calves and shins? Be smitten with knees
that creaked? Why didn't I worship
the dirty kitchen floor, clean it on hands and workable
knees, rock climb, salsa dance?

My disease raises its head and solemnly asks the same
questions and I want to smack this betrayal
of all things manageable—using an escalator, turning
over in sleep, standing to stir spaghetti
sauce, raking red maple leaves, wild sex.

In my scooter, I could trail my leg brace behind me
as a sea anchor, sail down mall halls,
wave at those too slow to keep up. "Whee," I'll yelp,
halting the contraption to gape at skinny-leg
jeans, red high heels, bikinis, knowing that before this new
life I never wore them and wonder why not,
why ever not.

–Marie Kane

Survivors in the Garden, Marie Kane, Big Table Publishing, 2012

What Not to Say to Me Now That I am Crippled

Try not to tell me to *take your time* when holding the door; if I could lag behind by choice,

I would (sluggishness is not an option with MS) and I appreciate that my sometimes

blind left eye discerns your kind face ignoring my conspicuous left foot drop, and that *do*

good is your mantra, but refrain from suggesting that I will walk well by

complying with these cures: a hysterectomy, or its opposite—pregnancy—or by the

repeated sting of honeybees, or by sipping Aloe Vera juice at a bank-account-emptying

spa at Versailles to enable my question mark spine to become an exclamation point, moreover,

should I ask for a bathroom, never, ever tell me that I can wait, and for the life of me,

do not cry out "Good for you!" as I relate my recent successes (as if I were five and had just

learned how to tie my shoes)—when I walk, stand, or stay awake more than I thought

I could ("Good for you!")—drive my car to physical therapy ("Good for you!")—shower by

myself ("Good for you!")—publish poetry ("Good for you!") and, when you spy me on my motorized scooter, don't saunter by and claim *sotto voce* to my husband, "I

need that more than she does," nor should you whisper that your mother, father, sibling,

next-door neighbor died of MS, but that I look Fantastic! Delightful! Splendid! Your

flood of words insists that I am a marvel; my doctors say I am doing well, considering.

–Marie Kane

Poems for the Writing, Prompts for Poets. Lynn Levin, Valerie Fox, eds. Texture Press, 2013. Reprinted with permission of the author.

Marie Kane's poetry is widely published in over twenty-five journals and four anthologies. Her chapbook, *Survivors in the Garden* (Big Table Publishing), largely dealing with MS, was released in 2012. Kane is the 2006 Bucks County (PA) Poet Laureate and the poetry editor for *Pentimento* magazine. See more at www.mariekanepoetry.com.

Dichotomy of the Tube Slide - A Case Study

(On Limitation)

SM: So I'm going to start this. I had a bit of an odd night last night and I'm sure it was kind of noticeable today. I seemed a little out of it. I got into my REM sleep, maybe around 2:15 or so I'm guessing, judging by the time I woke up. I started having this dream that I was at a café. It was a multi-story building and I was with Dianne, and we went up towards the top floor where they were allowing people to go down this long, enclosed slide.

DM: A tube slide.

SM: Tube slide. So Dianne went first and I went in behind her, and we were going down and we were going down, and then suddenly she ran into somebody and then I ran into her. So there was a backup in the slide.

DM: That's my worst nightmare.

SM: It's a total nightmare, and it turns out that there was a large man who had gotten stuck at the end. Whether it was because of his girth or because the end of the tube slide was a bit tapered, causing him to get stuck.

DM: Right.

SM: Didn't matter. I mean, it happened. So while they were working to free the man down at the bottom, there was like 37 people backed up in this long tube slide. It woke me up. Not because I'm particularly claustrophobic but because this is something that's happened to me maybe four times since I was diagnosed.

DM: You've been caught in a tube slide?

SM: No. I wish. It would be so much easier that way.

DM: If it's four times, then yeah. You'd figure after time two, you'd be like, oh, tube slide, fuck that.

SM: That's assuming I have control over my subconscious mind.

DM: Oh, yeah. Okay. Well, if it's a dream. Okay, sorry. Carry on.

(On Unification)

SM: And I'm glad to help them with that. I think that's a special thing.

DM: Right, and for whatever reason, folks want to be in print. I think that's part of that legacy. It's part of that, 'I was here.' It is a big deal that we're more than just our jobs or our collection of shit or loves or disappointments or whatever. There's this other thing. There's this animating force.

SM: Well, and it helps supersede the MS.

DM: Right, because it's generative. It builds instead of destroys. That's a way of fighting back, and it's a way of not giving up, not rolling over. Changing your diet is a way of not rolling over. Stopping drinking is a way of not rolling over. Or starting drinking. Those of you who want to start drinking, go ahead.

SM: There's no evidence to say that drinking obscene amounts of alcohol doesn't help.

DM: Get yourself good and liquored up.

SM: Give it a shot. You can even try heroin if you want.

DM: Right. Really? But yeah, the idea of building something is, I think, huge. And whether that's foundational or somewhere above that, but again, it lays a good bunch of work for other people to build upon, and at the same time opens all these sort of different conversations. Like what is this? What is this? How does this work? Not everybody's experience with MS is the same. Like you said, everybody's different. Everybody's path is different. Everybody's slide is different, and all the other brothers and sisters out there who have other diseases, chronic or not, that are working their way through whatever it is, seeing that there are these folks that are building something.

(On the Future)

SM: Well, all right. Back to the dream again. We're still in the dream. We never left the dream. If I'm in the tube and I'm constantly moving.

DM: If I'm in the tube.

SM: If you're in constant motion, the idea that you're in a tube, it in itself becomes like this infinite world. So there are no walls, per se. But when you stop, it's jarring, and one would tend to panic if the norm for you is this infinite space you're moving through. So it's hard to find that place of calm, and especially if I get to the point where I have to use a walker or a cane or into the chair eventually. Will I still be able to draw on that? I would think so, because over the course of time it becomes a practiced art. You rehearse it every day. So I would like to think I will know my lines well, when the time comes. Because I don't know if that time's going to come.

DM: Well, don't you? I mean, won't that come?

SM: Maybe. Maybe I'll be in a chair. Maybe I'll never need one. Maybe I'll just have this really pronounced limp. I don't know. I go with the assumption that I'll need a chair at some point. I start with that.

DM: So there is no script, I guess.

SM: No, it's different for everybody. The only thing that's universal is that it sucks balls.

DM: I can understand the ball part, having sucked a couple balls myself.

SM: Oh, yeah. I've been there. I've been on that ball ride.

(On Parenting)

SM: Let me go back to family for a sec. How do you think Mom's doing with all this?

DM: Who?

SM: Mom. Our mother unit. The one who birthed us.

DM: So what? You were saying something about how do I think Mom's handling this or dealing with it?

SM: Yeah.

DM: I think it's got to be really hard.

SM: Now are you speaking as her son? Or are you speaking as a parent as well?

DM: As a parent. The last thing that you expect is for your kids to be sick and to get some sort of chronic disease, or die before you. I think that specter, in the same way that you said that it caused you to sort of snap out of a malaise of sorts. It probably caused her to snap out of a similar sort of. . .

SM: Like this is all going ahead as planned?

DM: This is great. They're still alive. I've done my job. It's hard. So I think that she knows two distinct sides of this, and 100 different other ones. But the one is of the medical professional who knows the ins and outs of the industry research and how. . .

SM: It's interesting that you say industry.

DM: Yeah, and how diseases work and how families deal with grief or acceptance or whatever. I can understand that. Then there's just the raw, sort of, I'm your mom. She's great. She's scared.

SM: I'd be a liar to say…if I didn't say I was scared. But I'm far more interested to find out where this is going to go.

DM: Right. You don't get the luxury of not having MS, you know, in that way to say that. It sounds a little flip, but in a sense, it's left for everyone else to sort of figure out where they fit in that. Like it seems like you've been given this thing, a gift, a curse, and your reckoning with it is a daily thing. But for a parent, the only other thing I can relate it to is when it first hit me that I was – well, it's a long story.

SM: Well, yes and no, because at some point – and this is part of the dream as well – they started sending butter and olive oil down the tube. Shouldn't that be down at the bottom somewhere? Somebody's going to drown if you start putting that in there.

DM: Here's a salad. Well, still, you're in the best position. Because it's the people behind, it's the being in the middle. So that's interesting. You're the last one. So it is, it's very much, I mean, you're the captain of that boat essentially. Okay, going on. Let's take the metaphor out of the slide into the boat. So yeah, I mean, how do you widen that out so everybody's included? That's difficult.

(On Writing)

SM: Well, it's the Venn diagram times 20.

DM: Yeah, exactly. A great friend and wonderful writer, Martin Espada, is always curious. I sort of think of Martin as one of the finest American poets, I mean, straight up great poet. And on Martin's books and reviews of Martin, they're always like, one of the greatest or one of the fabulous Puerto Rican American poets ever, you know? It's like, okay, that too, but it's always hyphen American, you know. What about white American? You never hear that. Like, one of the best white American poets. One of the best Anglos out there. It's usually a white man. One of us white men. It's like our finest woman, you know. So how can everybody gain access to that non-hyphenated writer …

SM: Well, and like we talked about like Sontag and tuberculosis back in the day, that those people were considered enlightened or special.

DM: Right, and let me go further with this. It was thought of – the romantics. If you were a good romantic poet, you always had like a dwarf in your garden, someone to take care of, the wild man. I'm taking care of the wild sprite in my garden. You know, those folks were often sort of not the healthiest folks. But they thought of it as keeping the wildness of nature close by their lavish houses.

So I guess that rush of sort of – that life is so tenuous and so precious, and any upending of the easiness of life, of your life, of your living, of your expectations, then causes this whole artifice that you thought you were enacting or acting out to shatter. All of a sudden I'm alone in the vast and empty wilderness of MS-dom is as ridiculous as you're special. It's like no, man, you just go with it and you try and figure it out. Sometimes it's going to suck and sometimes little victories will happen. If you're able to build something on that, that's – again, as an artist, that's where it's at. So living the lie, sort of like, always be happy, is not acknowledging that you're stuck in the slide. There's a lot to be unhappy about if you're in a tube slide or in a diving bell or airplane. I hate sleeping bags.

SM: Like mummy bags? Or like sleeping bags at all?

DM: Sleeping bags with like – especially when the kids jump on you and you're in a sleeping bag. I'm like, all right, I'm going to throw up. Get off.

SM: Yeah, so you know what MS is like.

DM: I've been there, man. I try and stay positive.

SM: Welcome to my small group of 2.5 million people.

DM: 2.5 million people? Is that in the world or in the U.S.?

SM: Globally.

DM: Right on.

SM: Select group.

(A Diagram of Adjustments)

SM: Let me ask you something. What has it been like watching your brother over the last three and a half years? Does it seem very obvious that I'm progressing?

DM: Well, seeing as how I diagnosed you.

SM: That's another story.

DM: No.

SM: In fact, that will be a footnote for this.

DM: I diagnosed him.

SM: And we'll explain what that means. I'll get all DFW on you. Footnote, footnote, footnote, footnote.

DM: DFW? No, to me you're just an asshole.

SM: That's never going to change.

DM: That's always going to be there, whether you start walking with a cane you're in a chair. I'll still make fun of you. You'll still make fun of me.

SM: When you stop making fun of me, that's when I'm going to get worried.

DM: Right.

SM: That's when I'm going to think, oh my God, my brother has cancer.

DM: Yeah. Well, to be honest, the biggest drag – and I don't mean to bring this conversation down.

SM: No, not at all.

DM: But the hardest thing for me is that I know you and that we have a history, right? We've been around each other for a little bit.

SM: We've been in each other.

DM: We've been up in each other. But my kids, you know, they're getting to know you. They know you. You're great. But when we were at the Getty Museum and Ruby was maybe five or six, and Harlan was maybe two or something like that. We were doing a little chasing game and you couldn't run very well. This was before you were diagnosed, and I remember you saying like, man, my legs are weird.

(On Happy Faces)

DM: So everybody is dealing, I think, with their own struggles in one way or another, to come to this place to have two healthy, married children who are with good partners. Partners who love and respect them. That's a whole lot.

SM: I can put on a happy face with that. I'm not necessarily going to do it for MS, because I think that omits the whole other side or other facets of the disease. I can't be happy face all the time. I just can't.

DM: Well, that's the happy face thing that we were talking about, somehow finding that peace there, finding that strength or that will.

SM: But I think a chunk of that has to be embracing all facets of the disease.

DM: Right, the sucky parts as well as . . .

SM: The sucky parts as well as tiny victories.

DM: Yeah, so it can't be just, oh, what a blessing. I have MS.

SM: Right.

DM: Yeah, well, I mean, there's a whole population of people that call folks with disabilities special. They're special. And that specialness is a way of removing any sort of personality of the disease, positive, negative, in between. Oh, you're special. You know, it's like, well, no, I'm a whole lot more than that.

SM: That's like saying you're beautiful on the inside.

DM: Right, exactly. We use these words to not – and we were talking about this outside, but the whole – I mean, if you break down the word disease, it's two words. Dis and ease.

SM: See, but that's funny because it's one of the things that I can tell you about and tell mom about, or tell Dianne about, but you'll never fully get it and the way your brain has to rewire itself to process stimuli. Because everything comes carrying much more weight, and it's just harder to process it because of that, and slower.

DM: Well, and it struck me when we were in Maine, when you guys came to visit and we were on the rocks.

SM: That was the tight shorts, though, I think.

DM: Were you wearing tight shorts?

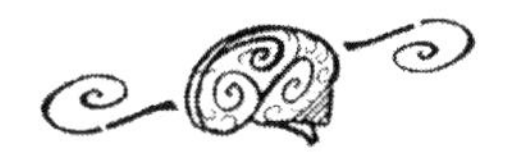

(On Engagement)

SM: That's getting edited out.

DM: Really? Shit. No. You're here more than just to sort of fuck hot chicks, if you can. And that's so sad. Like we were at that bar, walked past that bar.

SM: That was just weird.

DM: Yeah, that was just sort of – wow, really? This is what it all comes down to?

SM: Well, it was funny. We're coming out of the theater from seeing Inside Out, the children's movie, into what the children eventually become. It was a weird disconnect. It was like, you're not that. Who took over for you? I mean, you're not anger. You're not sorrow. You're not envy. You're just like somebody who was in the background and never seen in the movie. You're like self-pity or something?

DM: There was a whole lot of sorrow.

SM: There was a whole lot of sorrow, but Sorrow had her use.

DM: But masked, masked like, we're having a good time. But yeah, you know, the ability to feel something and to create conversation, and to create dialogue is what it's all about. That's part of that creativity. That's part of that why we're here, and why we're here is we're supposed to talk to each other. There's a philosopher guy, a French guy, who I taught this past year. Lobina – I can't think of his first name for some reason. Emmanuel Levinas, maybe? But his big thing was the ability to know yourself, and his idea was that we are all sort of responsible for each other. I cannot know myself, who I am, if I don't know who you are first. Only you talking to me allows me to understand who I am. So I have this responsibility to do the same thing for you, to engage you, and I can't know myself until I know you. In this dialogue, we find this sort of responsibility.

So we're responding to each other, and we're also responsible for each other. It moves you so far beyond the me, me, me thing. Like, I can't even know myself unless I know someone else. If the someone else isn't present, like the disability folks or whatever, then I can't know myself engaging with them, and they can't know themselves engaging with me, essentially.

SM: No, I totally buy that, because we touched on that already. After the diagnosis, the fire is lit and I started sending stuff out and getting published. Then it kind of stopped at a certain point. I thought, you know, what's wrong? Does everything I do just suck now? Or is there something else I should be doing? That's when it became more about 'outward' and creating this dialogue, asking other people to join me in this writing project.

DM: Right. It's like what Mike Watt says after every concert still, is, 'Start a band. Do your own thing.' If you don't like the music that's being played, play your own damn music. Figure it out. Again, you won't say that to everybody. For some folks it's a lot easier than other folks because the structure is already in place. But part of the responsibility again, of everybody, is I think start your own goddamn band.

–Sean Mahoney

Sean J Mahoney (SM) lives with his wife, her parents, two Uglydolls, and three dogs in Santa Ana, California. He works in geophysics. He believes that punk rock miraculously survives, that Judas was a way better singer than Jesus, and that diatomaceous earth is a not well known enough gardening marvel.

Daniel Mahoney (DM) is the author of *Sunblind Almost Motorcrash*, a book and cassette project published by Spork Press. He is in love with the train and the woman who fills the sky. He teaches at College of the Atlantic in Bar Harbor, Maine.

Decisions, Decisions

I tried to catch some fog. I mist. -Anonymous

One of the gazillion frustrations of life with multiple sclerosis is trying to explain "cog fog," also known as brain fog.

I once had a neurologist tell me that if I can't explain it, then it must not exist. Even in the brain fog moment that I happened to be in at the time, this comment didn't seem to make sense.

Isn't that the very point of brain fog? It makes things hard to think.

It also makes things hard to decide.

So even though today my brain is the foggiest it's been in a while, I decided I would take a moment try to describe "cog fog."

See what I mean about decisions?

One cognitive difficulty for me is simple math. Math was never my deal, MS or not.

All I remember about my high school math classes is that one teacher was always covered in chalk dust and the other took points off if you turned in a page ripped from your notebook that still had the little squiggly pieces attached from where you ripped it.

MS can make me easily overwhelmed and every factor imaginable takes over when trying to decide something or trying to do basic math. Another frustration of "cog fog" is that it can often frustrate others, especially when I need to combine it with numbers and decisions.

Here are some things that my MS brain makes difficult in my life and that are hard to explain to those who find it weird.

Making coffee — This should not be a big deal as I don't even drink coffee. Put some hot water and a tea bag in a mug and I am good to go for the day.

The problem comes when I have to make coffee for someone else. Many people have tried to show me how to do this and I can never remember the coffee scoops per water ratio.

Sure, I could write it down. But where? How will I remember where I have written this information down?

One might suggest that I just read the directions on the back of the coffee container. But those directions offer variables- for stronger coffee do this, for a larger pot, do that.

How do I know what is a large pot and if my guests want their coffee stronger or weaker? Why can't they just drink tea like the rest of the world?

Multiple email addresses — Whenever someone changes their email, or gives me a second or even third email address, I'm lost. Not to mention the fact that my email server keeps changing the rules.

So what do I do? If I have to send an email I will send it to all the addresses I have for the person. This causes them to get several emails and get annoyed with me. I'll ask which address to use and they will send a response like, "this one, this one's the best."

Well which one is that? My computer just puts your name in the address bar so I still have no idea which is your preference.

Or, to get back into the decision thing the person might say "I just use this one for work," or "I just use this one for fun stuff." Now I have to decide if what I am emailing is fun or not and then go back to trying to figure out which email address is which.

Keys — My dad recently picked up my key chain and wanted to know why I had so many keys and what were they all for. I had no idea.

I started to try to figure it out and just got overwhelmed. One clearheaded day I actually started locking and unlocking stuff to try to further investigate. And then I got confused again.

I went to the hardware store and bought those little color tabs you can put on keys to signify where they go but of course, I can never remember which color is for which lock. I can write that down but where- on my keys? That certainly would make it easier for the burglars.

Gratuity — The best example how brain "cog fog" can mess with an MS'er is tipping.

Generally I'm a nice person who wants to be generous. I waitressed one miserable summer and even though I was super klutzy and lousy at it, (I choose to blame that on MS even though it was 20 years before my diagnosis,) I appreciated a good tip. And I'm not cheap.

But if I go to a restaurant with someone the words I dread are "I'll get this, why don't you just pick up the tip?"

Why is this tough? First you have to remember the going tip rate- 18%, 20%, 25%. Then you have to do math.

Then you may want to account for the variables associated with a range from lousy service to wonderful service.

(I may be nice and I would never stiff a server but if you are rude you are getting the minimum tip: unless of course I screw up which is likely.)

Then, because it's not cool to leave change, you round the tip off-more math. And more decisions- should I round up or down?

To help combat this particular frustration I got myself one of those tip cards. So if I'm in the tip paying position I will pull out my little card. And it helps, if I can read it in the dim light of the particular establishment I happen to be at.

But often, my companions object to the card.

"You don't need that to figure out the tip- just round off the bill, take 20% and then lower it slightly. Oh wait, he was really nice, raise it a bit. Do you have enough singles? It's not cool to leave change, even quarters. Oh wow, that's a really generous tip, did you mean to leave 40%?"

It's enough to make someone never want to go out to eat.

But the confusion doesn't end there. It pops up again with hairdressers, taxi drivers, delivery people, the kid who pumps your gas, and on and on….. I swear I gave my hairdresser a 60% tip last week. No wonder she loves me; it has nothing to do with my wavy hair and sparkling personality.

In the grand scheme of life, none of these cognitive difficulties are that big. And when you put them in the context of the grand scheme of multiple sclerosis, they're even smaller.

But still, when you need a way to describe what can't be described, here you have it.

At least, I think this is descriptive.

I can't really decide….

–Yvonne DeSousa

Portuguese Soup with an MS Twist

It was a privilege growing up Portuguese, especially when it came to Portuguese food. Portuguese delicacies are awesome.

What? You don't believe me?

Trust me. I have way too many extra pounds on my 5'3 frame to prove it.

We Portuguese folks have our own veggie soup and even I, the self proclaimed arch enemy of vegetables, love it.

Of course, my ancestors taught us right; we load our veggie soup up with sausage so it doesn't taste like a veggie soup.

But it totally is! It has carrots, potatoes, onions and kale, the super food of my people.

Some people put tomatoes in their soup to make it even healthier and the soup also has lots of beans which offer protein and fiber. I'm telling you, this soup is good stuff!

And depending on how involved you want to be, there are many different ways to make it. Some people go all out, growing their own veggies, raising, slaughtering and smoking the pork themselves and soaking the beans for days.

Before MS, I actually learned to make this soup and I must say, it came out pretty good. (I personally didn't slaughter anything though..)

But no matter what the experts say, cooking with multiple sclerosis is hard and shortcuts are often needed.

So I was thrilled to discover a recipe that made the soup process much easier. Instead of using salt pork for flavor, (I have bought salt pork before but don't know what it is and am not sure I want to know) it uses bean and bacon soup. Soup for your soup? How incredibly convenient! Many Portuguese people I know would disown me for using this version but we just won't tell them.

The problem was, I needed even more shortcuts. Chopping and peeling are particularly hard for me and so I dared to wander down the canned veggies aisle of the supermarket and was thrilled to discover that potatoes and carrots come in cans! I scooped them up.

That meant I would only need to wash the kale- take it from a Portuguese person, you really have to wash the kale well. It's so good that bugs just can't resist it. Now if you are cooking broccoli for some strange reason you probably don't need to wash that at all. It's so gross even dumb bugs stay away from it — chop the linguica (mine is a linguica family, I think the chorizo people are from the islands) and chop the onions.

Well, one onion. Chopping onions was really hard for me and so I only use one in my version. I knew I was saving myself a ton of work.

Mid-afternoon I started washing the kale. Washing kale should not be that tiring but when you have MS, everything is tiring. Since I needed to stand at the sink, my legs started to ache during the washing process. I set the kale aside to dry and then rested for a bit.

Next, I opened my cans of veggies. But with weak, achy fingers, that was an exhausting task too. And so I rested some more.

Next I started to slice the linguica which wasn't hard at all. And since by then I was pretty hungry, it was a fun chore. Slice, snack, slice, snack — oh this slice is uneven, better just munch on it now.

I hadn't even started cooking the soup yet and it felt like I had been working on this recipe for days instead of an afternoon.

I saved the worse task for last- the onion. I pulled out the sharpest knife I could find, which is incredibly dangerous even in the best of circumstances. Not the wisest move when being used by somebody whose hands have a tendency to randomly drop stuff and throw things across the room.

I sat at my kitchen table and carefully started to chop. I have never been good at chopping onions the right way and have even watched cooking shows for tips. Nothing has ever worked.

Soon my eyes stung and wouldn't stop tearing and drastically uneven pieces of onion were scattered all over my table. There had to be an easier way.

This soup was good for me, mostly- the sodium and the sausage not so much- and I was making the easiest of the easiest of versions and yet I was still struggling.

Why does everything with MS have to be so damn hard??? Even a recipe I have been making for years and watched my mother make for years before that.

As I whined about the miserably chopped onion and felt sorry for myself, my phone rang. It was a dear, supportive friend who asked what was going on. I told her my frustrating plight. She had good advice,

"Yvonne, there's no reason for you to chop onions if they give you such a hard time. You can buy them frozen, already chopped."

Her advice was spot on. So spot on that I remembered hearing it before. My mom had told me that many times. So many times that it occurred to me that I might just have bought……

Sure enough, with my friend waiting on the phone I opened my freezer to find a bag of frozen chopped onions, lying on top of a bag of frozen, prewashed kale; bags I had bought when the cooler weather had first started me craving my favorite soup. Now my MS frustration was no longer about how I am not even able to chop an onion and get exhausted just rinsing fresh kale, but how it's hard to even remember the shortcuts you have already designed for yourself.

But, ahhh the soup was good, even with the canned veggies. And the next time I make it, it will be even better with canned AND frozen veggies.

That time for sure, it won't take too much out of me. And, well, if it does, luckily kale soup goes great with Portuguese wine.

Even luckier, another dear, supportive friend bought me an electric wine opener!

–Yvonne DeSousa

Yvonne deSousa uses her sense of humor to defend against the MS beast. She has published the well reviewed memoir, MS Madness! A "Giggle More, Cry Less" Story of Multiple Sclerosis, and writes a weekly chronic illness humor blog. You can contact her through her website, yvonnedesousa.com.

Cicadas

Aerial assembly, looming in lofty arboreta -
Rhythmic, symphonic, yet shrill in sound -
Summer's siren - high in pitch, a vibrating trill -
A conclave…a warning, or is this worship magnified?

Constant, clear in tempo...somewhat pleading in tone -
Music composed by the dutiful male -
An insect to squash would squelch, mislead
The purpose of humid dusk and
Curtail nature's short lived euphony.

Summer begs - it calls for cicadas to appear -
A life and purpose unlike other winged creatures -
Comprehend, compose, they communicate such
Mysterious secrets we'll not know -
Random - fleeting is their raucous existence -
Without caveat or anticipated memorial they disappear
Leaving behind an odd, deafening silence, until
Life moves on to resume the familiar.

In ripening months, when cicadas come, engage -
Reflect and appreciate a guttural concept of performance -
Contemplate purpose, unique and always changing -
An evolutionary life-force, audible even after departure -
A mortality, never truly finite...instead,
Cyclical in its renewal - when summer begs.

–Mary Pettigrew

PTSD

Like clockwork, panic wakes me with a start -
My body, mind and soul at war again
Spanning decades, this solo battle leaves me
Broken, breathless -
Exhausted, sweat drenched nightmares
Find me in the darkened haze - I pause
Until I'm urged to get out of bed -
Wading through the deep abyss of sleep deprivation
I splash cold water on my face - some relief -
Looking into the mirror, I examine scars external –
A surgeon's signature leaves
Visible wounds, healed like "tattooed tales" -
But my eyes…whose eyes are these?
They're silently screaming, revealing
A hidden myriad of stories blocked, painful years lost -
Invisible, overlooked by all who know me, yet I now see
The internal infection of toxic damage -
It's there – and in my eyes you'll see the pain -
I'm still bleeding - and quickly
Running out of gauze.

–Mary Pettigrew

Obstacles

As of late, I'm stumbling into ditches -
Potholes, sinkholes numerous and constant -
Sludge filled blockades swallow me up,
Re-routed attempts to
Destroy my plan - my path.

Though tiresome, I succeed to claw
To climb out of each ditch –
Wash off the filthy muck and mire -
Weakened mind, body and soul, yet
Somehow, determined to grow stronger.

That's all I can do…what I'm supposed to do -
Never allow monstrous, muddy obstacles
Opportunity to overtake, to win –
Instead, revise and draw a new map –
Alter the route, and continue the journey.

–Mary Pettigrew

Mary Pettigrew is a late blooming writer from Texas who specializes in creative writing. She is a 1990 graduate from The University of North Texas. Mary was diagnosed with MS in 2001. In need of therapeutic outlets, Mary discovered that creative expression gave her new purpose, passion and life.

If the People Stare, Then the People Stare

Imagine a thick fog, you can't see anything around you, it's so thick and overwhelming. You are unable to move, you're stuck you're even afraid. You feel lost without the help of those around you, you wonder where they are? Now imagine that you are blamed for having gotten lost in this thick fog. You should work harder to get out! It's not so bad you just need a little motivation to get out! These things are easy to say from afar, but not very helpful whatsoever while you are in the midst of this fog.

People with Multiple Sclerosis will know what this feels like. Being misunderstood hurts. Being misunderstood because of your illness hurts even worse. I am used to being misunderstood or looked upon as different; I have bright pink hair that tends grabs people's attention. Other than my hair I look like your average able bodied young adult woman. However, what cannot be seen by others is that inside my body is not cooperating with me. Others look at me and see no difference. They, those others, become agitated with me and they don't believe me when I tell them my legs are in severe pain or why I cannot maintain my surroundings. It's hard to prove to others what they cannot see. MS gives us so little energy to work with, and trying to plead our case takes a significant portion of that energy away from us. With misunderstanding comes a sense of feeling alienated and a sense of being different, ostracized, and not like everyone else.

Have you ever felt weird? Of course you have, everyone has at one point or another in their lives. September 2012 changed a lot for me. That is the date I was diagnosed with Multiple Sclerosis, in my mid-twenties. As far as I could remember I've had neurological problems, yet no doctor would listen to me. Hypochondriac is what they would think. But they were wrong. The diagnosis came as somewhat of a relief, for the first time I was validated and my doctors now treated me with respect. This was newfound and strange. Because they would now listen, from then on I would be sent to many specialists to try and figure out what's wrong with me. I experienced that same hurtful condescendence from doctors that I was all too familiar with in my life.

Since my official diagnosis I've acquired quite a few new diagnoses. With being diagnosed with MS, and later many more diagnoses, how do I not feel weird? How is it possible to live like anyone else my age – because of course they will not understand. I was thrust into a new world of illnesses, prescriptions, tests, doctors, and despair. This was a personal journey, because no one truly understood.

Having an illness or disability can make anyone feel alienated from their peers or may make us feel weird or seen as not *normal* or like those around us. Yes, I do embrace being different. But I have struggled to accept that I have a chronic illness and that this chronic illness makes me 'different'. My pink hair makes me ‘different’ but neither of these things makes me weird. The only thing that makes me “weird” is me labeling myself weird.

There is nothing wrong with being different. With things we cannot change, we must accept even though we struggle. There have been times that I’ve had severe vertigo, to the point I literally looked intoxicated and people would stare. There have been times when I walked into a store and people stared at me and thought that I’m a criminal because of my unique choice of hair color.

I’m pretty used to being misunderstood; my life has been a constant unconventional existence. I have always seen being different or a little unusual as a good thing. My unique hair to me represents not worrying what others think of me. I had this distinct hair color before I was diagnosed. It has given me the strength to not worry about stares or comments from people. It’s helped me become a stronger person. It has given me thicker skin. I’ve learned a great lesson by looking different; I get both compliments and confusion. But that’s okay. One could say that the same goes for being disabled. Some people with MS will be stared at with confusion or even with disdain for needing assistance when they don’t look the part.

With a disability come stares. When a person sitting in a wheelchair suddenly stands up those around may gasp and whisper of how these people in the wheelchair are merely faking! “Wow!

They are using a wheelchair but can walk!" they say in anger and prejudice. People need to be educated that disability means and looks very different than the classic preconceived notions. Many people with MS need that wheelchair because they *know* they need to conserve that little precious energy it takes to walk from here to there for another important situation.

At times there are aspects and symptoms that come from multiple sclerosis that others simply do not understand, and you can try your hardest to explain to those around you how they affect you or your life. But many will refuse to understand or say they understand but truly are looking down on you. They may see you as simply lazy, "Why can't you clean your floors, it doesn't take much effort!" they tell you when they visit, they cannot grasp that this simple task may come easy to them but to you it would take a great amount of energy to exert. With MS you have to decide which activity deserves that precious energy you contain and which do not.

At the airport I am in need of a wheelchair to go through security. Why? Because the energy exuded during this whole process is enough to put someone with MS in extreme fatigue and leave them unable to function for the rest of their day. Traveling is exhausting enough for people without an illness! Looking different is hard enough, a wheelchair itself may make us feel different or make us feel a wide range of emotions from feeling defeated to feeling as if we are not allowed to have this accommodation because of how we look.

The various feelings that may arise from the fear of looking or feeling different are hard enough, but what if that person has something that makes them look *too* able bodied? What if that person in the wheelchair is wearing heels? So what! Yes, you will more than likely get a number of hateful stares, but if needing a wheelchair in order to be able to use heels for an important event is what you need then so be it. If there are stares, then so be it, those around you may not understand your struggles, or understand that you want to feel normal just like everyone else. If it means using a wheelchair as needed, then by all means, allow people this choice. Accommodations are hard to ask for and they are hard to accept, it's natural to not want to look or feel different.

Yes, I know it is not easy, but it is worth it. The example of wearing heels is merely an example from a wide range of scenarios. I wish to demonstrate with this example that taking a chance and being different or looking different is hard, however we must remember that those around us or society are *not* allowed to dictate what you wear or do not wear because you are diagnosed with a chronic illness or have a disability. We must conjure up all the strength it may take to not allow those comments or stares to affect the way we live our lives and we cannot berate ourselves for wanting to be how we choose. Being a relatively young person diagnosed with an illness is an immensely difficult situation. Not only must you come to grips with "what ifs" of what your future holds, but also "what ifs" about what your present life holds. I am a person who thrives from going to concerts; it has been one of the only things to bring me life. When I was diagnosed it was as if I no longer felt able to attend one; I no longer felt normal or felt like my fellow peers. I was gripped with fear of being inside a crowd, because of my balance and painful legs I felt as if I no longer had the luxury. That I would no longer be able to see close up the bands that I so adored. I felt weird.

I would in the past always arrive early to concerts to make sure to secure a good spot near the stage; I am no longer able to do this. So because a person has a disability does that mean they now need to be confined to disability seating? Does that give other people the right to choose? I have been fortunate enough to have great experiences from simply *asking* for accommodations. I used to feel as if I was cheating others… but you know what? I wasn't and am not. They have the luxury of arriving early and standing hour upon hour, I do not. I no longer am able to take those risks, it has now become dangerous. So if simply allowing myself to ask for help and in that way I'm able to be just like my peers and fellow concert attendees then once again, so be it! I have been fortunate with getting understanding help from staff, but that cannot be said about my fellow attendees. I have gotten snide comments, people making sure that they ask rudely where the disability seating is for me, so that I don't take their spot. Here is where that thick skin comes in. Here is where that risk of looking or feeling different comes in. And they must come to understand that not all illnesses or disabilities are visible.

I have struggled with this idea since being diagnosed. But the realization came to me one day. I can't. I can't convince these people, nor do I need to. It's as simple as that. I do not need to tell them what is wrong. I do not need to tell them why I need special accommodations. I do not need to tell them how these symptoms affect me daily, why I can't clean the floors, why I can't go out, or why I had to cancel plans. I don't *owe* them that.

Being different is hard. Getting stares is hard. But it's how one approaches being different that truly makes the difference. It's how we ourselves approach these differences that makes, well… the difference. We can choose to hide or we can choose to take the accommodations that are available. If we choose to hide our pain and discomfort to look normal, what we are really doing is being uncomfortable so that others aren't uncomfortable.

It's okay to take accommodations and it is okay to simply ask for help. Stigma and fear of what others will think or say of us should not hold us back from living a fulfilling life. If others choose to belittle us or treat us badly that is a reflection of them and not of us. All that is in our power is to keep our heads held high and continue living our lives.

Being misunderstood is challenging. Trying to explain yourself is exhausting. If they stare then they stare. It only affects us if we let it. We are not weird. We are only weird if we define ourselves as so. A disability can make us different but it does not and will not make us weird.

So I began writing to not only document and share my MS story, but to also prove to myself that I am more than a diagnosis. To see what I'm capable of with these diagnoses. I have more to offer than just MS. I am not an illness. This illness does not make me weird or abnormal. A disability can make you look unique or different but we cannot change these aspects of ourselves. It's our approach. It's how we find that inner strength and thick skin to not allow the stares or comments from others discourage us. I want to show others in a similar situation that we are not our illness.

We are not weird.

–Marissa Perez

Marissa Perez, aka Peeks, is spirited and strong-minded. She aspires to be a writer. Shy yet extroverted she's never afraid of challenges and new experiences. She's modeled, avidly attends concerts, and has a bachelor's degree in Psychology. Having led a life of adversities, she's kept her good-nature and determined attitude. http://www.peekies.wordpress.com/

Serendipity

"I deal with people with MS every day at work. I don't want to come home to it."

Harsh words for a 26 year old to hear from the man she thought she was going to marry. People say that if you want to know who your friends are and who really cares about you just wait until you either get married, pregnant or sick. This bit of insight became clear to me after ending up in the hospital after waking up from a nap with crippling vertigo, double vision and profuse vomiting.

I lived with my boyfriend Joe who was an emergency room nurse at a local hospital. He came home after his hour and a half workout to find me in the bedroom refusing to open my eyes as the vomiting became more intense with every passing moment. I had managed to call my oldest sister Melissa over and tell her that something wasn't right and I needed to go to the hospital. Joe started asking my sister questions, trying to piece together the picture we were painting. My sister went on to explain how I had been diagnosed with optic neuritis two years earlier. At that time doctors had told me I had a 50% chance of developing MS and my sister now thought this might be the start of something serious.

Joe, being that he was a nurse, did not believe this to be true. "She just needs vitamins and Gatorade. She'll be fine."

They took their conversation downstairs and away from me as my sister did not want to upset me. They went back and forth about what they thought would be best for me. My sister came back upstairs and was visibly angry when she asked me if I was comfortable enough to have Joe take me to the hospital. I said that I was and she left.

The vertigo was so intense by this point that I really felt like I couldn't walk. I felt as if my body just quit on me without so much as a two week notice. I begged Joe to carry me down the stairs and to the car but to no avail. This was a 6'1", 250 pound man that spent every free moment he had in the gym. He was solid muscle and probably the strongest man I knew, but he wouldn't carry his 5'2", 100lb sick girlfriend down the stairs. It took 45 minutes for me to get down those stairs, scooting my butt down one step a time as I clutched onto the garbage bin like life support. I stopped to vomit on each step. Fifteen steps later I made it to the car.

The ER doctor was looking at me sitting in a wheel chair, barely speaking, vomiting and stating that I could barely walk. I no longer resembled the confidant, carefree woman I was when I moved to Colorado a year and half earlier but rather a hunched over, jaundiced version of myself. With his brows pushed together in puzzled thought he said, "I don't get it. You're a seemingly healthy young 26 year old and you're telling me you can't walk all of a sudden."

"I have optic neuritis," was all I could manage to say and I watched as this registered in his mind and his face dropped.

"I want to try something. Stand up and walk towards me."

I gripped the arms as I slowly rose from the safety of the wheel chair. Once I was convinced that I wouldn't fall face first onto the lovely emergency room floor, I did as I was instructed. I took three steps towards the doctor; three steps that looked like a baby giraffe first discovering it has legs instead of a healthy twenty something year old. Falling onto the bed I hysterically asked, "What is wrong with me?"

The next several days are a blur. A blur of IV's, MRI's, spinal taps, wires and injections. The doctors were thinking it might be an inner ear infection, Lyme disease, Multiple Sclerosis or possibly a brain tumor. They ran tests, one after the other, to rule things out. I had no clue as to what they were leaning towards until they did the lumbar puncture at my bedside. It was a pediatric neurologist that was on call that day and he wanted results he could see. He gave me a sedative and prepared my back to begin the spinal tap. I jumped once at the initial needle going into my spine before settling into a sedated state of mind as he drew the cerebrospinal fluid from my spinal cord. He was disappointed when the fluid appeared to be negative for MS. To me this was great news! All I kept thinking was please let this be an inner ear infection. Please, let this be fixed by a strong dose of antibiotics.

Please, let this be a false alarm, a fluke a mistake. For days I wondered when they would reach a conclusion. We had done several MRI tests and I was anxious to hear the results. Please, don't let it show any lesions, was all I could think.

During this time my sister Melissa made sure to be by side every chance she got. If she couldn't be there she would ask my friend Ryan to sit with me. Ryan and I became friends about 2 years earlier after being introduced by my brother and although there was a mutual attraction it was something we didn't talk about. He came to see me on his lunch breaks and after work, sitting with me for hours on end while we watched funny yet mindless YouTube videos. He gave me a blank "get well card" and said he would sign it later.

One day while he was visiting with me I needed to go to the bathroom and at this point I couldn't get there by myself. I pressed the button to call the nurse into the room to assist me. In walks a male nurse with ginger hair who looked like he was in his second year of high school.

"I need to go to the bathroom."

His eyes shifted from side to side as he pointed at Ryan and said, "Well he can help you."

"I don't *want* him to help me."

The nurse helped me get out of bed and let me grip onto him for support as he walked me the couple feet to the bathroom. I was drowning in the hospital gown, one size fits none, and told Ryan not to look as the back of the gown left nothing to the imagination and I was wearing hot pink underwear. He assured me he would not look.

The nurse left me in the bathroom and after a couple minutes I realized that he was not coming back.

"Hello?" I called out into the oversized bathroom as I listened to my words ricochet off the walls.

"Yeah the nurse left," Ryan stated from behind the door.

"What?! Why would he do that? I told him I don't want you helping me!"

Silence.

I was beyond embarrassed at the thought of my male friend (who I secretly found attractive) helping me off the toilet and back into bed. Ugghhhh!!! With my face scrunched up in agony I asked if he would open the door and help me?

I was standing and holding onto the handicap bar next to the emergency assistance cord when he entered the bathroom. We smiled uncomfortably at each other as he offered his arm. I latched onto him as we made our way back to the bed at a snail's pace. I was trying to hold the back of my gown closed as well as hold the front from hanging open as I ungracefully climbed back into bed and quickly threw the blanket over my unshaven legs. I was so mad at that nurse and I made a mental note to tell him.... if he ever came back.

I was in a relationship with Joe and there was talk of marriage on the table. But once I was admitted to the hospital and was no longer the fun version of myself we all began to see a different version of Joe. You would think that dating a nurse while having a huge health scare would be helpful but in fact it was the opposite. He came to see me at the hospital a couple times, texting on his phone the whole time and staring at the clock. Once he put his twenty minutes in he was out the door. He was not present the day the doctor told me my fate.

My sister, brother and Ryan all sat with me in the hospital room as the doctor walked in prepared to give me some answers. He asked if I would like anyone to leave before he began, at which point I stated no. My heart was racing and beating though my chest as it does when I recall this moment in my life. My palms were sweating and I tried to appear calm. A dry lump hung in the back of my throat.

"After looking over your MRI results we're lead to believe that you have what is called Multiple Sclerosis."

I covered my face and began to weep as he continued, "You have eight lesions on your brain." After that I could no longer hear anything he was saying. If you look up the definition of Multiple Sclerosis you will find exactly what he said. To me it was all white noise.

After several moments the doctor gently asks, "What are you thinking right now?" My sorrow quickly turned to rage as I screamed, "I'm thinking about how I want to have kids and not be in a fucking wheelchair!"

There were mumbled apologizes and hugs as everyone excused themselves, leaving me with my angry thoughts. Ryan squeezed my toe on his way out, not knowing what else to do. How was this happening? This isn't even in my family. I'm too young to have something wrong with me. I just took a nap. I took a nap. I TOOK A NAP!

My mind became a black pit where positive thoughts go to die. Who's going to want to marry me now? How will I get a job and explain how I can't use my left arm right now but hopefully someday I can? How am I going to have kids and explain that mommy is too sick to play right now? What if I have a baby and then relapse? How will I handle a newborn and a relapse? What if I can't pick the baby up? What if my arms are too weak and I drop the baby? Can I still breastfeed? I'm going to have to live in a ranch house so I don't have to go up and down stairs. How much does a wheelchair ramp cost? This diagnosis put a huge fear inside me when thinking about the future. The "what ifs" were endless and draining.

The day I was released from the hospital and returned back home Joe yelled at me about the housework not being done. A week later he started telling me I was lazy. When I needed an epidural blood patch after developing the worst headache of my life following the lumbar puncture, he told me that he was a nurse and had never heard of such a thing therefore it was not a real procedure. He wouldn't take me to the hospital for my steroid infusion because the football game was on. We got in a screaming match and I wasted what little energy I had. I went to stay at my sister's house.

I sat on the living room couch as I explained to my family and Ryan what had been going on between me and Joe. I kept my sunglasses on as I tried to shield my face and hide my tears. My symptoms had worsened since being released from the hospital, probably due to all the stress, and I couldn't even walk 5ft without a walker. I was having muscle spasms that caused uncontrollable pain to shoot through the entire right side of my body. It would start with my right hand working its way down my arm then picking up at the top of my thigh and painfully sliding down my leg and through my toes. The pain would take my breath away, making me cringe and cause my right hand to curl up as if I were trying to flash a gang sign and lift my right leg off the floor all at the same time.

Everyone told me to go lie down and try to get some rest but I was too weak to use my walker to make it to the couch in the neighboring room. A smiling Ryan pushed a computer chair with wheels on it in front me.

"Hop on. I'll give you a lift." His gentle blue eyes reassured me and we laughed as he wheeled me away.

Melissa and Ryan took turns watching over me. They would make sure I ate, took my medicine and kept me company. The pain was excruciating and nothing was helping. The only thing that distracted me was Ryan and when he would leave I would cry uncontrollably as I was more aware of the pain when he was not around.

An excruciatingly long month later I was finally on a medication that helped calm the muscle spasms. I was able to once again move my limbs the way I wanted to and without immediate pain. I returned back to the house I lived in with Joe and tried to move forward but things were too far gone with us. I spent all my time with the dog outdoors and he spent his time drinking with his buddies at the bar. Before I got sick we would talk about a future wedding almost daily but once I was no longer the fun party girl version of myself it became "we'll see". We had become roommates instead of two people who loved each other and saw a future together.

My sister tried to make me see that things weren't working out and that I should leave the relationship however, her way of making me see things her way was to yell them. I did not respond well to that and, although I knew it was true, I instead became defensive and came up with excuse after excuse as to why Joe was acting the way he was. Part of me didn't want to hear it and part of me didn't want to believe it. I wanted things to return to the way they were before.

The one person that was close to me during this time was Ryan. Our friendship had grown over the past few months and we talked every day now. If I complained about something to him he would just listen. He never gave advice or his opinion, he just listened. He became someone I trusted and turned to often.

One cold April night Ryan and I met for dinner at a little sushi place on the south end of town. We sat at the bar and ordered Sake and spicy tuna rolls. We made small talk and caught up before the conversation turned to my relationship with Joe. Ryan began to calmly point out things that I didn't realize while I was in the hospital and a drug induced state. He pointed out how awful he had been treating me during the past few months and again I began to defend him. But Ryan gently persisted and continued to open my eyes and force me to see what everyone else had been seeing for months. I was dating an asshole.

It was clear what I needed to do but fear quickly showed its face and made me scared at the thought of having to explain my new situation to a potential partner.

"It's not that easy. I don't want to explain this to every guy I meet because nobody is going to want to deal with this."

"That's not true."

"Yes it is. People won't understand."

"Yes they will."

"Who the hell is going to want to date me?"

"I do."

I raised my eyes to meet Ryan's and he wore a handsome crooked smile. I was so taken aback that I had to ask, "What?"

"I care about you so much and with everything that has been going on, it makes me care about you even more. I want to be with you. I love you." Ryan crossed the friendship barrier and put all his cards on the table.

"I care about you too," was all I could manage to say as a smile so big it hurt my cheeks took over my face.

Going through the experience I had really made me open my eyes and see what an amazing person I had in front of me all along. After we began dating he filled out the empty" get well "card he had given to me that day in the hospital.

"I've never met anyone quite like you, so I don't even really know what to say. You are my best friend. You make me smile every time you walk into a room, yet at the same time I get so nervous that I sometimes don't know what to do. You give me this feeling that I've never really felt. I can't describe it exactly. I just know that I want to always be there for you and always take care of you if you'll let me. Old and grey means old and grey."

On August 23rd, 2014 we were married. Sometimes your life ends up being different than what you had planned, and sometimes it is better that way.

–Katie Roberts

Katie Roberts is a patient coordinator for a plastic surgeon. Originally from Chicago she moved to Colorado and was diagnosed with Relapsing/Remitting MS in 2012 at the age of 26. She enjoys volunteering, hiking, writing and spending time with her husband Ryan and their two cats Figaro and Luigi.

Church

The church at the end of my street has its own TV show. Not TV like primetime broadcast, but TV like channel 978. And it's not, strictly speaking, the church's show. The church is always in the show - the outside on the titles, the inside for the rest - but apparently that doesn't make it the church's show. The pastor says it's the congregation's show. But it seems to me that the congregation, like the church, is just a thing that's in the show, and that they get, probably, less screen time and space than the building itself. The pastor told me that I have a strange way of thinking about things. Which struck me as a strange comment, coming from the pastor of a church with its own TV show.

I think *he's* strange — the pastor. His forehead is furrowed, and the furrows extend right over the curve at the top of his skull. His dog-collar hangs out stiff and sideways. And he lives with a monkey. It sits at his table and presses its face against the glass of his bay windows, with both hands flat on the glass.

Maybe it's the monkey's TV show, really. He's the star. The monkey is there to show how the Bible is right. The pastor takes it to places and insists it's his relative, then they film people's reactions.

The first one, they took the monkey to a restaurant and filmed it smashing up the table and screeching at the other customers.

Then when the manager asked them to leave, they filmed him and the pastor in a two-shot and the pastor insisted that the monkey should be treated just like any other customer. The manager declined the invitation and offered to call the police. Then they show that on the show and the pastor he says after it that that proves it: no way we're related to monkeys - they can't even eat a lasagna with a knife and fork.

It must have gone over well, because, like I say, they did a lot more. The pastor rang up airlines and told them he needed a seat for his relative and they said OK. Then he told them it was a monkey and they said he'd have to go in the hold, they couldn't have a monkey running around the cabin. And the pastor said, but he's my relative. And they said, no, he's a monkey. And the pastor came on the screen and said, that proves it, see? Darwin was an asshole.

He didn't say 'asshole'. But you could tell he wanted to.

It went on for weeks. Pastor took the monkey to all the local businesses and demanded service. He wanted his monkey to take tennis lessons, get a haircut, join a gym. They all said no. I thought the monkey looked disappointed.

I asked the pastor about it, and he said he thought it was the best way to prove to people that no-one really believed in the *theory* of evolution. I said I believed in it.

The next morning, the pastor shows up at my place with the monkey and the cameras. Wants to rent a van. I said, sure, no problem, does your relative have a credit card? Turned out he didn't, so the pastor had to use his, but that's fine I said, no rule against that. Does your relative have a driving license? Monkey didn't have one of those either, but I said no worries, we'll just put it under your name. Pastor looked a little more furrowed than usual, but he signed the paperwork and I got him his van. The monkey looked pleased, climbing up into the cab of that three-and-a-half tonner. I got him a cap from the office with the name of my firm on it, and he seemed happy about that too.

C'mon Pastor, I said, patting him on the shoulder. Start it up for him.

–Scott Whittaker

Scott Whittaker is a scrimshanking philosophunculist, an argle-bargling blatherskite, and a bloviating apple-knocker. He often struggles to find applications for his collection of ostentatious words.

Charity Skydive

It was a bright summer day, so the signs were ominous — the charity tandem skydive would go ahead. So with some degree of apprehension we set off for Chiltern Park Aerodrome in Oxford.

And, there followed a wait of some hours, to really build up the tension. But, at last we were called forward and given a run-through of what, and what not, to do and we were introduced to the men and equipment that would, hopefully, bring us back down to earth safely. To be honest, it didn't seem likely that anything could go wrong!

Well, having been loaded onto the plane, somewhat unceremoniously, we slowly ascended up to a height of 10,000 feet. And, that's quite high! The door was opened and three solo sky-divers moved towards the open door and proceeded to throw themselves out. That was quite surreal.

Now, it was my turn. My cameraman went out first and......... climbed alongside the plane, to film my exit. It just seemed a ludicrous, crazy thing to do, but I wasn't scared!

We launched ourselves out of the plane and proceeded to take up the regulation spread-eagled sky-dive posture. That was fine, but 10 feet in front of me was a cameraman, falling on his back, recording whether I smiled or not. I don't think I let him down!

All too quickly, the parachute was opened and my free-fall came to a very abrupt end. And, then we slowly drifted back down to earth, where we were met by the ground personnel, who ensured that a safe landing was made.

And, the question that you are always asked on landing, "would you do it again?" Well, yes, I would, subject to a couple of conditions. One, don't make the harness too tight. I lost the blood supply to one arm on the way down — I suppose it was better than potentially slipping out of the harness. And, two, when the parachute is opened, don't twirl me round in circles — I don't do roundabouts!

But, I'd done it. Another tick in one of life's boxes. And just a dead arm and a bit of sea-sickness to show for it! It just had to be done.

–John Wiltshire

John Wiltshire is just your average 50-something teenager, with the physical attributes of an 80 year old. MS came to call on him some 30 years ago and, just like an uninvited guest, has outstayed its welcome. This wasn't part of his life plan, nor his wife's or his two sons. But it sure keeps life interesting.

Interview: Cyndi Zagieboylo

SOOM reached out to current National Multiple Sclerosis Society President Cyndi Zagieboylo for some friendly coffee talk, chit chat, and banter.

SOOM: Thank you for taking the time Cyndi. So you've been president of the National Multiple Sclerosis Society for almost 4 years now. How did you get started with the Society in the first place? Do you have a personal connection to MS?

CZ: I started college with the general sense that I wanted to do something to improve the world. I was inspired by people who choose to be positive about life and I wanted to know what I can do, what we can collectively do, to support people in finding a positive path.
I didn't know anyone with MS when I started my MS Society career 30 years ago. Much of what I have learned about living my best life is from people affected by MS.

SOOM: "...a positive path." I like that. Do you do any other volunteer work outside of the NMSS?

CZ: In addition to being an event participant (current fundraising event is the MS Challenge Walk on Cape Cod. 50 Miles -- All Smiles is my team, in case someone wants to join) and donor for the National MS Society, my family is involved in community clean-up projects (including an annual responsibility for 2 miles of our street). When my children were growing up, my husband and I coached teams, taught Sunday school, and prepared and served meals at a soup kitchen. Also, we sponsor a family every year at Christmas time.

SOOM: Wow – hats off to you and your family. Do you enjoy getting out to the local MS Chapters when you can?

CZ: I travel throughout the country and I appreciate meeting people in the MS movement wherever I go.

SOOM: Is there an international component to the NMSS? Does the Society interact with their counterparts in other countries?

CZ: Oh yes, the National MS Society is the largest MS organization in the world and we have a very important role in the MS International Federation. In fact, our founder, Sylvia Lawry, helped to found the International Federation, so it is a very important part of our fabric. The National MS Society funds the most promising research in the world; we've always had an international presence. Our most ambitious international activity at the moment is the International Progressive MS Alliance. The National MS Society, USA, is a founding member of the Alliance, which was formed in 2012 to speed the development of treatment for progressive MS by removing scientific and technology barriers and focusing the world on the gap in treatments for people with progressive MS. There are 10 countries represented in the Alliance, plus the MS International Federation, and more are joining.

In addition, we play our part in building capacity in fledgling MS Societies around the world. We receive requests from other countries and we do our best to be supportive.

SOOM: That is really encouraging – especially for all our progressive kin out there in the wilds. Do you have any plants in your office?

CZ: There is a plant in my NY office. I'm not sure who waters it.

SOOM: Does said plant have a name? I ask because we have a Fiddle-Fig plant in our home that we named Felix. It just seemed like the right thing to do.

CZ: It's a spider plant, I know that much, and I appreciate it, but I have not named it.

SOOM: When you have a day, or days, off, what can Cyndi Zagieboylo be found doing?

CZ: Mostly, I love to be with my family. My husband and I ride a tandem—mostly on off road trails--and we like to go to the gym together. I enjoy cooking—especially when the 4 of us (I have two sons, ages 20 and 21) can be together.

SOOM: Off road on a tandem bike? Now that is especially adventurous.

CZ: Not really, there are many rails to trails in my part of New York and in places we travel. It's not exactly exciting—more nature-filled, peaceful and relaxing. There are times we go on a 35 mile ride and see only a handful of people.

SOOM: Is there a particular cuisine you are drawn to?

CZ: I love food! There's not much I don't enjoy. For "comfort" food, I'd go with Italian. This past weekend I made great fish tacos!

SOOM: Yum. If salsa could be reclassified as its own food group I would be ever so happy. So where do your musical tastes run? What do you like to listen to for work? For leisure?

CZ: I like the sound of quiet. I don't play music when I am on my own, but I do enjoy listening to most other people's preferences.

My neighbor plays a soft jazz that I can hear in the summer across our yards—that is pleasant.

SOOM: Agreed – quiet is nice. And beneficial. What are you reading these days or is there even time for recreational reading?

CZ: At the moment I'm reading a biography on Howard Hughes—he had an incredible life and tremendous impact on our lives today.

SOOM: What are your thoughts about Hematopoietic Stem Cell Therapy (HSCT) specifically and stem cell therapy protocols in general? Do you believe, as many do, that they indeed do contain the promise of MS eradication?

CZ: It's so important that we use the scientific method to test hypotheses. There is hope in stem cells, and research is needed to understand the potential of stem cell treatments. We must be careful about forming "beliefs". Scientists, especially, need to be skeptical, to question, so that we can continue to add to the body of evidence toward solutions.

SOOM: So true. There are a handful of folks out there crying "Cure! Cure!" but we must keep in mind that this is a very young science. I for one am glad that the vast majority of medical practitioners are moving forward slowly and with confidence. Any thoughts about new studies involving Biotin or N-Acetyl Glucosamine?

CZ: I'll defer that question to our research experts.

SOOM: Fair enough. Would it be too forward if I were to ask a legacy question? What sort of legacy do you hope to be remembered for at the Society?

CZ: It's hard for me to think about being remembered for something—we have so much yet to do and I want to be part of all of it. I am proud to be part of the MS movement and I believe that, together, we are changing the world for people affected by MS. I hope that people know that I care deeply; that I will not look away from the most challenging problems. The National MS Society exists because there are people with MS and we want to do something about that. We want to achieve a world free of MS.

SOOM: You have been more than generous Cyndi. Thank you so much for taking the time. I wish you and the Society continued success.

Cyndi Zagieboylo has served as President and CEO of the National Multiple Sclerosis Society since 2011. She received her bachelor's degree in rehabilitation counseling and psychology from Springfield College, followed by a master's degree in social psychology from the University of Connecticut. She lives in Honeoye Falls, NY.

Sean Mahoney conducted this interview on behalf of SOOM.

Revelation

Revelation in a tear
of salt and memory…
Who she was,
but can't recall…
Dreams that cease to be

Horse and rider conquer
a river full of life…
Dry her up,
make her forget…
A husband and a wife

White, and red, and black…they come
Earth beneath her quakes…
They chase away
lost picture books
of memories, as she wakes

Send a dragon…Falling stars
Seven angels singing…
She waits for you
Oh palest horse,
Waits for what you're bringing

–Judy Crowe Olsen

Mirror Song

Can I love
the skin on my neck,
that hangs,
like a tired linen curtain…

Eyes shadowed by a year of fears.

Chipped teeth
that shift in my mouth,
Restless sleepers.

My mother's hands… a mother's hips
These lines that deepen around my lips…

that sing goodnight
to who I was…

And whisper… can I love?

–Judy Crowe Olsen

Shy Bear Pass

How far will I carry a bottle of Ale up a mountain trail?

Halfway to the peak (that is not a peak), I open it. To share with thirsty mosquitoes… and my funny cousin.

The one with two-tone hair, who makes me laugh so hard I stop climbing to pee. And swat the biting flies without falling over.

Is it her, the ale, the altitude? Or the forest, full of thirsty spirits that want to share my laughter.

A fat marmot turns his nose at my sweat, while a pair of chipmunk cousins chases each other, giggling, across a log.

A rabbit stops on the trail ahead, standing on his hind feet with his ears erect, he is nearly 3 feet tall. With a disdainful twitch of his nose, he is gone.

At the peak that is not a peak we drop our sweaty packs. The bugs have grown tired of our ale-laden blood.

We write a poem in the guest book and make a list of "things you do not want to be caught saying when a room gets quiet." We are never quiet. And Shy Bear will only watch us from his hiding place.

Maybe he will come out later, to lick the sweat from this spot where we rested against the great Cedar. A tree that we touched and said a silent thank you for its patience.

Maybe Shy Bear is laughing now, and reading our poem to the rabbit.

–Judy Crowe Olsen

Judy Crowe Olsen lives in Washington State, works full time in Environmental Health, and actively supports NMSS. She loves to hike, write, drink tea, and spend time with her two sons. Diagnosed in 2003, she turns to nature for physical, emotional and spiritual health. Judy shares her writing at www.justonlyjudy.com.

Nurturing Kids & Fighting Lesions

Before I became a mother, my rosy and naïve opinion of parenthood was best summed up by this passage from the Book of Psalms: "Children are a gift from God". As far back as I can remember, I practiced what I was certain would be spectacular mothering skills on unsuspecting baby dolls, somewhat offended cats, and (when appropriately supervised) the occasional human child.

My confidence lasted precisely until May 26, 2004, when I laid eyes on my first son after an emergency C-section. Fast forward 11 years, 3 boys, an MS diagnosis, and a painful divorce, I've decided to hijack the sentiment Thomas Paine wrote in 1776 about the tumultuous American Revolution—"These are the times that try (wo)men's souls!"—because with minimal modification, it provides a 21st century application for the scope of life, parenting ***and*** neurological diseases!

The moment I saw my MRI one fateful day in March 2010, it was immediately clear that I would need to re-configure my plans--every single one of them--beginning with something as basic as food, because I was still nursing the son I'd given birth to just 3 months before. There was a substitute for feeding my baby, but not for slowing down the disabling of my central nervous system. MS had been lurking for some time and in the "medically necessary vs. medically beneficial" debates between lesions and breastfeeding with my wonderfully supportive neurologist, the lesions ultimately won.

This was simply the first of hundreds of parental adaptations I've encountered in the five years since. It's a truth well-known to those with a neurological disease that *having* fatigue is exceeded only by the exhaustion of *managing* it. Who among us hasn't asked "What should I make for dinner tonight?" but instead, "What should I make for dinner tonight (at the last minute, of course) because suddenly my right leg won't hold me up and let's not even *discuss* what's been going on with my bladder today..?!" The symptoms of MS, difficult to manage for anyone, become an even more frustrating burden when it siphons the very energy parents require to remain active and engaged in our growing children's lives.

Since my children's father left our home in August 2014, and the divorce ending our 14-year-marriage awarded sole custody to me, I've become even more acutely aware that although I find many physical responsibilities of childrearing terribly difficult to perform and painful to endure, I have no choice but do them. It's been well-worth the struggle to maintain my sense of humor, because often, it's what the four of us have most needed to adjust to what I call our "newest normal".

The day my oldest son went to get some juice for his brothers and called out, "Oh, for crying out loud, who left the rubber mallet in the fridge--***again***?!" was yet another tender reminder that my memory has become increasingly problematic. But knowing the boys were watching my reaction, instead of weeping in frustration, I burst into laughter. I remarked how I was pleased I'd clearly improved upon the time I left the ice cream sandwiches on their dresser… for nine hours… in July… We then launched into a round-robin of increasingly bizarre and hilarious predictions about the kinds of "MS Easter eggs" they might find in the upcoming years.

I'd like to think that had I known MS would be an indiscernible 4th child (always demanding attention, constantly making messes, and permanently living under my roof), I still would have had the audacious courage to become a mother. It is my absolute belief that having a chronic disease has made me a better parent; less focused on my boys being on the "best" travel sports team and more in-tuned to their individual personalities and needs. I tell newly-diagnosed parents there's nothing wrong with using the adversity their kids are growing up with as a means to strengthen their character—to use the illness as an example of determined resilience in practice--rather than provide a convenient excuse for potential weaknesses. I try to encourage them to remember little eyes are watching how they respond not just to their disease, but to life in general—while there's nothing wrong with grieving the truth my kids have a parent with MS, and this means they know and witness difficult realities their more carefree friends are spared—because let's face it, nobody comes out of life "unscathed" of challenges.

And while I refer to them as ***my kids***, I've always been well-aware my primary job as a mother (regardless of an MS diagnosis) is actually preparing them to be ***men***; the type who can rely on their resilient character when the inevitable "times that try men's souls" require them to be flexible. I believe because this has always been my goal, the traumas the boys and I have experienced in the last 5 years haven't even come close to breaking our collective spirit!

With each of the limitations my MS progression has imparted, I've determined to adapt and function at highest capacity I can, although the fight to remain independent and maintain a positive attitude has taxed the limits of my patience, energy, and self-esteem every time. There's nothing more frustrating than sending my two oldest boys to get dressed for school, but instead hearing them descend into a violent scrum in the upstairs hallway (because one of them tried to wipe a booger on his brother) and I have to use my limited energy to haul myself upstairs to sort it all out, when we're already running late! But that's the unpredictable nature of parenthood—and really, folks, that's also the unpredictable nature of ***life***.

So I encourage well-meaning people to not feel sorry for my sons—those lucky boys have been provided the perfect training field for a successful life: They are being nurtured by a chronically ill but fiercely jubilant mother.

–Emily Rhoades

Emily Rhoades is a recovering history nerd, avoidant housecleaner, and eternal optimist. She lives her crazy wonderful life in Peoria, Illinois with her 3 sons, 2 cats, and 1 MS diagnosis. You can follow her blog at lesionedlife.com.

My Magnificent Spirit

"You never know how strong you are… until being strong is the only choice you have."

— Cayla Mills

"Character cannot be developed in ease and quiet. Only through experience of trial and suffering can the soul be strengthened, vision cleared, ambition inspired, and success achieved."

– Helen Keller

They say you don't know yourself until you suffer adversity. If that is true, and being diagnosed with multiple sclerosis is the biggest adversity I have been through, then what I know of myself is I am a magnificent spirit.

Before being diagnosed my life looked great. I had a successful career, a loving husband, and a great house. I did what I wanted. I traveled, cooked exotic meals, tended an abundant garden, and made pottery I shipped around the globe. My life was full and grand.

My inner world was not so successful. I had bouts of depression. I was stressed all the time, wondering when something catastrophic was going to happen. I was a workaholic. My friendships were shallow and disconnected.

Yet my life wasn't bad, it simply wasn't fulfilling.

I am one of "those people" who found has found the silver lining in being diagnosed with a chronic illness. That diagnosis sparked a journey in which I saved myself and nourished my spirit. Today, six years later, I am fulfilled even as my life outwardly looks the same.

On that snowy December morning in the neurologist's office, of course, being diagnosed felt like the end of the world. In that moment, I melted. To make matters worse, I would have to give myself an injection. It was too much. I wanted to cave in on myself and run away. And yet . . . and yet . . .

In the millions of moments that have followed, I have learned more about my spirit, my character, my grit and who I am than I could ever imagine. I learned I am powerful, loving, inspirational and free. This is the story of my journey.

The Power of Choice

Why was I always stressed when I had a good life? Because I was living under the delusion I could control things in my life. I tried to control everything; my boss, deadlines, colleagues, spouse, and my fellow commuters to name a few. If you have ever tried to control any of those things, you know control is a game that leaves you bitter, overwhelmed, angry, cranky, miserable and stressed. Or maybe that was just my experience.

Either way, after the initial shock of being diagnosed with MS wore off, I knew I needed to change how I was playing this game of life. I knew I had to start with my health. For years I suffered from various maladies; everything from sinus infections to digestive issues and migraines to excruciating menstrual cramps. I was proud that I was so adept at knocking illness down like moles in a Whack-A-Mole game. I felt in control of my health.

The irony was not lost on me that I was diagnosed with a condition doctors don't know how to control. While my control freak was having a temper tantrum in the doctor's office, my inner power ranger, Wanda, with whom I was not yet acquainted, went to work, called forth to respond to the moment. As she did, a sense of calm flowed over me as I listened to my doctor run through my options. Wanda whispered in my ear "*you need to get off this hamster wheel of stress and control girl. You need to recreate your life. You need to create a new normal where control is not the goal.*" I had no idea who Wanda was or what she was talking about, but I left the doctor's office determined to figure it out. In that moment, I was just beginning to feel my true power.

After a few days of research, of the Internet and self-reflecting varieties, I realized the answer to recreating my life was to feed my control freak, not starve her like I had been doing. I had spent my entire life trying to control the uncontrollable and thus believed I could control nothing. Yet I was overlooking all the things I could control. It was time to make a different choice.

There were so many things I could control. I choose to build a pillar of wellbeing through diet. It turns out I had a library of nutrition books I hadn't really used. I dove into these books with the fervor of a cancer researcher. Four days after being diagnosed I had transformed my diet. I choose to forgo red meat, dairy, gluten and sugar. I know most people looked at these choices in horror. "What **can** you eat", I was asked. I will agree this new diet was not always fun but I never used willpower to stick with it. Instead, I choose something more powerful; I choose to make it fun. I discovered new ingredients and cooking methods and soon was enjoying desserts and to die for meals again.

The results of my choices have been impressive. I shed unwanted pounds, discovered energy I had forgot was possible and I have been symptom-free. My diet has morphed over the years as I learned more about my body and the disease. I now juice and blend my meals on the go, eat copious amounts of green leafy vegetables, use healthy fats and only occasionally eat grain. In a month, things could change because I am always using my power to choose what will make me feel my best.

My choices extended beyond my diet to include daily mindfulness practices, including being mindful of my language. A few weeks after receiving the MS diagnosis, I visited my long-time naturopath. When she asked why I came in for a visit, I said "I have MS." She stopped me.

"You don't have MS. Don't say that again. It is not yours. You simply have been diagnosed. The minute you own MS, it will be yours forever."

Here was another way to claim my power. I could choose how to frame my relationship with MS. I know this might sound like a semantics game or psychobabble, but language and attitude became another pillar of my new normal. To this day, I don't say I have MS because I don't. I've have never owned MS as mine. I have chosen to view MS as a label, one I won't wear. Some have told me I am in denial. I'm not. I choose to believe I am a spiritual being having a human experience. Yes, I get tired and have pangs of pain or trip walking to the bathroom. In these moments I wonder if some disease mechanism is at work. The truth is neither the doctor nor I know. So I choose not dwell. Instead I tap into my power by controlling what I eat, say and think. The rest does not matter.

What power will you choose to tap into today?

Returning To Love

Louise Hay, in her book "Heal Your Body" says the metaphysical root of multiple sclerosis is "mental hardness, hard-heartedness, iron will, inflexibility. Fear." Bullshit, I thought, when I first read her book. I wasn't hard of mind or heart. Yet my spirit snagged on the truth of these words just enough to give me pause.

While driving home from the neurologist that fateful morning, I kept hearing in my head:

Love it. Love the MS. Go home and find that book by Marianne Williamson. She will teach you how.

To this day I don't know the source of the voice I call Wanda. All I know is she spoke to me loud and clear. I sensed I better not ignore her.

I pulled my yellowed, dog-eared copy of "A Return To Love" from the shelf when I got home. I had read these pages at least ten years earlier. As I flipped through the book, I felt I had read it all those years ago in preparation for this exact moment. I searched for the passage I was sure was there. And there it was . . .

> . . . for a person diagnosed with a physical ailment, the call to change is imperative. . . the last thing a sick person needs is something else to hate about themselves.

She went on about the importance of loving the illness whether it was cancer, AIDS or MS.

How could I ***not*** *hate MS? How could I love MS? Wasn't MS going to ruin my life,* I thought. If not hate then what, I asked. At that moment, I was not prepared to love MS. I didn't even love life. How could I love this disease?

Despite being unable to see the way in those early hours, something deep inside me convinced me to trust Marianne. I would begin to cultivate love; if not for MS, than at least for my life. I began keeping a gratitude journal, writing down three things each day. I ventured into the world of vulnerability and started talking about my fears. I read, reached out and risked. I faced my fears and walked through them. Love began to blossom.

Returning to love was not as inward focused, as it might seem. I created safe containers for others to be vulnerable and soften their own hearts. In that I softened mine even further. I discovered all the beliefs I had (and there were many) that kept my heart hard. I learned how to break through them to create love for others and me. I shared my lessons with others.

As I opened up to my loving spirit, I began to love my life and eventually loved MS. I loved MS for what it made possible, including slowing me down, waking me up and focusing me on creating a purpose-filled life. I suspect Marianne Williamson knew this when she wrote those words; working to love the disease broke open love everywhere in my life. I discovered I was a loving spirit.

How will you choose love today?

Inspiring Others

I was standing in the kitchen talking with my husband about who we would tell about this diagnosis and when. I did not want to tell anyone. I didn't want sympathy and I didn't want to draw attention to myself. My husband, on the other hand, wanted to know if he could talk about the diagnosis while fund raising for his next MS Society bike ride. He also wasn't sure it was good for either of us to live under a secret. As we discussed the pros and cons of telling others, with me seeing more cons than pros, Wanda chimed in loud and clear.

"Of course you will tell others. You will inspire others. You will speak up and inspire them."

This time Wanda's voice was accompanied by a vision; a vision of me standing on a stage and speaking to thousands. I had no idea what Wanda was showing me. I had never inspired anyone. I thought people felt sorry for me because I worked so much. I was also terrified of public speaking. Wanda was clearly losing her touch, I thought.

A year later I stood in front of 10 people and gave my first talk. I spoke about the dangers of sugar. I was nervous, my voice wavered and I forgot a huge amount of my material. I considered the presentation a disaster. My audience, however, was inspired to try giving up sugar. Hmmm, a small victory for them, but a huge victory for me and my audiences to come.

Over the next five years, I spoke to audiences of a few hundred and wrote to thousands on the pages of my blog all because I learned to trust the voice of my spirit. Six months after extolling the evils of sugar, I stood on a stage at a National Multiple Sclerosis Society event in front of 75 people and told my story. Two years later I took the stage in front of 100 women to talk about creating a new normal. Each time my voice was stronger and more inspiring. Just about every week someone reaches out to me to tell me how something I wrote or said inspired him or her to change his or her life.

I write none of this to brag, but instead to inspire you to listen to your spirit even when it seems preposterous. I was petrified of public speaking. I thought I had nothing to say. Yet here I am living with purpose, living **my** purpose and none of it is about me. I speak and write to share what I've learned. The more I share, the more I see the truth of Wanda's words . . . I inspire.

How can you inspire?

Free To Be Me

As I have shared with you here, I was a prisoner of my own mind when I was diagnosed. I feared everything – losing my job, husband, or home – in any given moment. Everything was scarce in my life– love, time, money, and appreciation. I couldn't get enough to fill the void.

While it may sound like I was neurotic or a basket case, I was not. Instead, I was experiencing the human condition.

Fear plagues and imprisons us all. If you are willing to look, there is something you fear. It's a fear that dims the brilliance of your life as it did mine. I have seen how fear is an every moment reality for me; for my fellow humans. Sally fears dying alone. Becky fears being fired, because she "knows" her family will leave and she will be homeless. Kyle fears being abandoned and ends up sabotaging every relationship he has, recently pushing away the woman he loves.

Fear can be compounded for those living with multiple sclerosis.

> *What if I get a bad performance review because I'm more forgetful these days? Will I lose my job? What if I'm late again, will I get written up? What if I wake up and can't move tomorrow? What if my spouse can't handle it and leaves me, will I die alone? What if I can't find a new job?*

My fears didn't start with being diagnosed at 42, but started much younger, in response to hurt. I didn't get married until I was 38 because I feared getting hurt again. I worked long hours at work because I believed that is what it took to avoid rejection. Indeed, I had experienced rejection from my parents, teachers, and friends. I did not want to repeat that hurt.

I realize now – years later - I had not been rejected. Instead I had created an elaborate story to make sense of the hurt I felt in any moment. I had been living in this web of stories that kept me cocooned from the life I desired. I was a prisoner in a cell of my own making; running faster and faster on the hamster wheel, but getting nowhere fast.

Our fears shape our behaviors and begin to define who we are. We create stories about the events in our past; stories that help us make sense of our pain. We reinforce these stories and thus our fears. We make our selves unavailable and then wonder why our relationships end. In my case, I kept working harder so I would be accepted.

We think of freedom in political or financial terms. I am convinced we have it wrong. The most important form of freedom is personal freedom. Personal freedom is not given to us but rises from the rubbish left behind when we deconstruct our hamster wheel of fear and limiting beliefs.

I longed to feel free the day I was diagnosed.

During the last six years I have worked to dismantle my hamster wheel. It's been a slow process at times. In other moments, I feel as if I riding a bullet train. I am not finished. I still experience fear. But even in this fear, what characterizes my freedom is the ability to transcend the fear and live fully.

Would I have created my freedom if I had not been diagnosed? I have no way of knowing and it's not a question I spend much time pondering. What I know is on my journey, I have found freedom. In that freedom, I have found joy, purpose, love, inspiration, power and healing.

How are you creating your freedom today?

# # #

Multiple sclerosis is a challenge and a blessing. It sparked a journey of discovery and breakthrough. I have traveled from stress to hard-heartedness to loving. I give what I have to give and in this I inspire. I choose to control only that which I can control. Sure I slip up. But I no longer beat myself up, for I no longer pursue control or perfection.

I am not perfect. But I am a powerful, loving, inspirational free woman with a Magnificent Spirit.

–Laurie Erdman

Laurie Erdman is a writer, business leader and speaker on a mission to inject love into the way we live and work. She teaches audiences and readers how to ignite their lives with passion and freedom. You can learn how ignite your own life at www.LaurieErdman.com

Final Words of Inspiration

Life is precious, challenging, and worth getting out of it what you can.

Being a lover of American history, one of the items on my bucket list was to visit the actual trail of the Lewis & Clark expedition. I just returned from an RV road trip with my husband and brother to do this. During the trip, I reflected on the similarities of their journey and life with MS.

When Lewis & Clark began their journey to the Pacific Ocean across the continent, they went into unknown territory. Daily they encountered obstacles in the wilderness they had to overcome, and had to rely heavily on the support of each other/strangers, their skills, ingenuity, and creativity in order to survive and prevail. The team of thirty-three persons suffered; one died. They experimented. They documented. They learned. They managed and accomplished incredible hardships. There were moments of the deep despair and defeat, and moments of high joy and success.

They found their way. I found my way. You will find your way.

–Debbie Petrina

Reprinted with permission from *Managing MS: Straight Talk From a 31-Year Survivor, 2011*

Debbie counsels, writes, educates, researches, and advocates awareness and understanding of MS through her website www.DebbieMS.com, social media, and other activities to help anyone dealing with MS. She resides in Glendale, AZ with her husband, and enjoys reading, swimming and camping. Debbie has lived with MS for 35 years.

Be Part of the Change

We wait to be called on,
or at least we used to,
biding time until asked to contribute,
but no longer.

Can we afford to wait?
Too much is lost,
it's taken too long.
While accumulating more costs.

Relying on others, isn't working or
a valid excuse. They can't do it alone.
They shouldn't have to.
It's not a solo act,
We're all in this fight.

Something's gotta' change.
Speak up, opt in.
Opportunities are everywhere,
Don't just look. Act.
Advocate. Participate.
We can't afford to procrastinate.
Whatever it takes 'cause change is needed
And we need it now.
Step up.
Make it happen.

An Open Invitation

You are invited to be a part of the change for multiple sclerosis research through iConquerMS™, a patient led, patient centered online research project, where people with MS share their health data and their research questions.

iConquerMS™ is just one of several projects of the Accelerated Cure Project, the beneficiary of the proceeds of Something On Our Minds, Volume 3. You can learn more about the Accelerated Cure Project and join iConquerMS™, at the website www.acceleratedcure.org.

–Laura Kolaczkowski

Laura Kolaczkowski serves as the Lead Patient Representative for iConquerMS™ and is active in the MS community at the local and national level. She writes for MultipleSclerosis.net and maintains her personal blog at InsideMyStory.

INDEX

Allen, Angela

I Can Still 85
I Went to the Doctor 87
The Wheelchair Cruise 86
This Wretched MS and Me 84

Binns, Cherie

Invasion 46
Looking Backward ... Thinking Forward 47

Brown, Marcus

Loss of Independence 8

Carrillo, Albino

After the Seizure, 8/22/13, 1535hrs 3
Fire Escape 1

Chevalier, Constance

Finding Joy Amongst Pain 90

Crowe Olsen, Judy

Mirror Song 182
Revelation 181
Shy Bear Pass 183

DeSousa, Yvonne

Decisions, Decisions 136
Portuguese Soup with an MS Twist 141

Dolce, Kim

A Kiss before Falling: The Noir of MS 4
A Problem of Faith 27

Emrich, Lisa

Solace 73
The Mermaid in the Pool 74

Erdman, Lori

My Magnificent Spirit 190

Hopson, Ashli

New Beginnings Equal Happier Endings 70
The Dreamer 71
The Survivor's Anthem 72

Howard, Carolyn

Senryu Progression 12

Huff, Ronald

Every Step I Take 79
Loss of Independence 8
Rome Wasn't Built in a Day 102

Kane, Marie

Invocation 116
This Is The Life 118
What Not to Say to Me Now That I am Crippled 120

Kolaczkowski, Laura

Be Part of the Change 203

Kyriakou, Caroline

A Writer 17
In The Fight Together 18
The MS Walk 19

Mahoney, Sean

Dichotomy of the Tube Slide - A Case Study 122

Marissa Perez

If the People Stare, Then the People Stare 157

Milligan, B.

damn legs 26
Hunger 25
taking sides 26

Perez, Marissa

If the People Stare, Then the People Stare 150

Petrina, Debbie

Final Words of Inspiration 202

Pettigrew, Mary

Cicadas 147
Obstacles 149
PTSD 148

Rhoades, Emily

A Lucky Lady 20
Nurturing Kids & Fighting Lesions 185

Roberts, Katie

Serendipity 158

Sellman, Tamara Kaye

Ouroboros 13
The Broken 42

SOOM

Interview: Marc Stecker, Wheelchair Kamikazee 52
Interview: Cyndi Zagieboylo, ... 175

Stecker, Marc

Footprints and Shadows: The Tao of MS 64

Straiton, Brieana

Dancing with Multiple Sclerosis 105

Suri, Nidhi

Borrowed Time 34

Tierman, Brenda

Multiple Sclerosis 41

Whitakker, Scott

Church 170

Wiltshire, John

Charity Skydive 173

Made in the USA
San Bernardino, CA
08 December 2015